Recent Advances in Gout

Edited by Rie Kurose

Published in London, United Kingdom

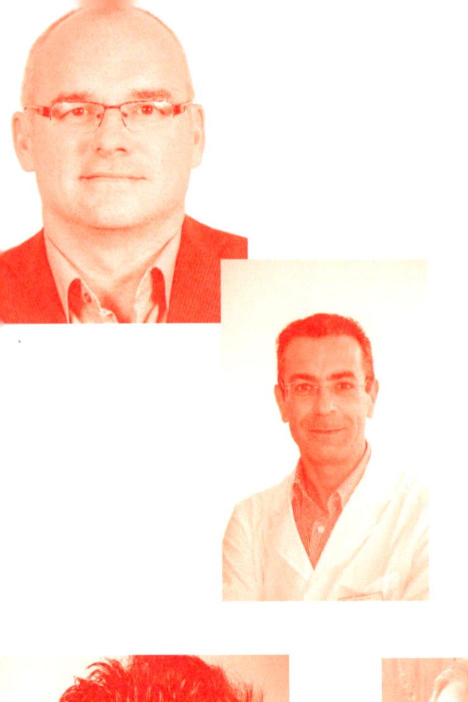
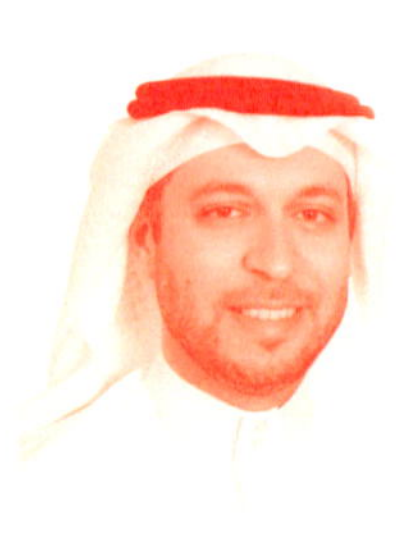
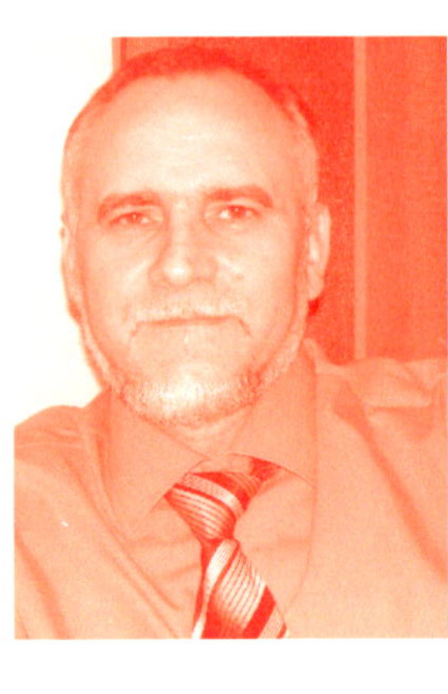
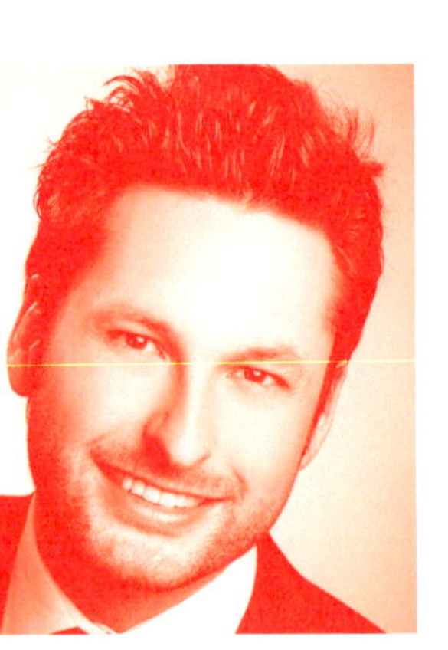
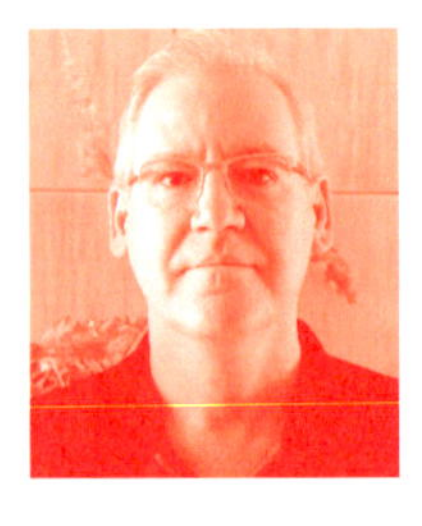
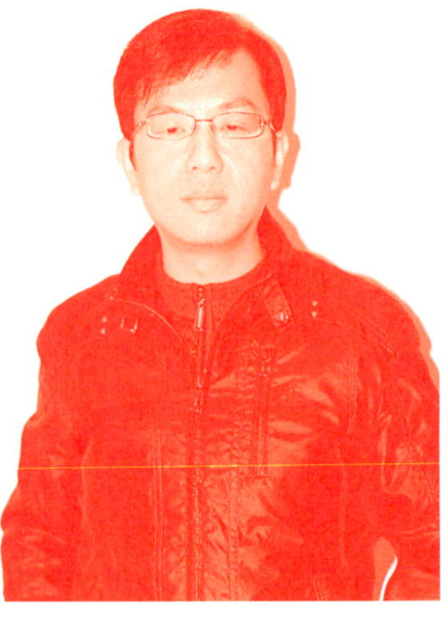

IntechOpen

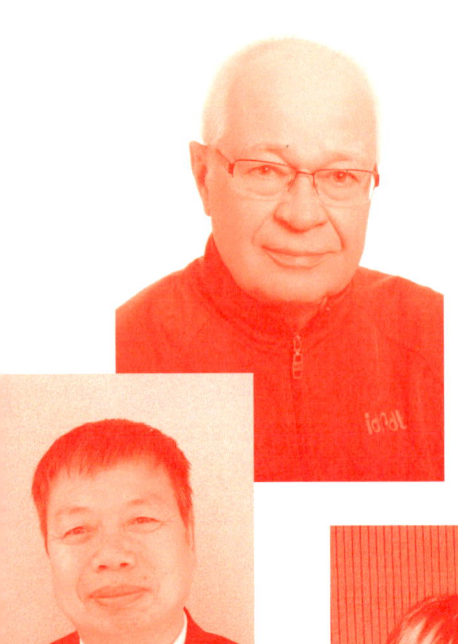
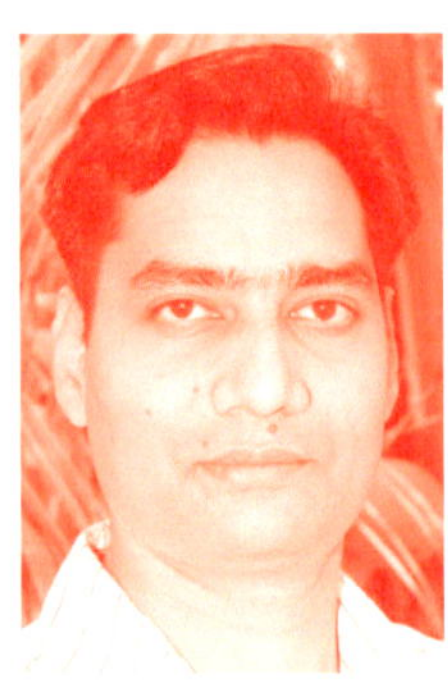
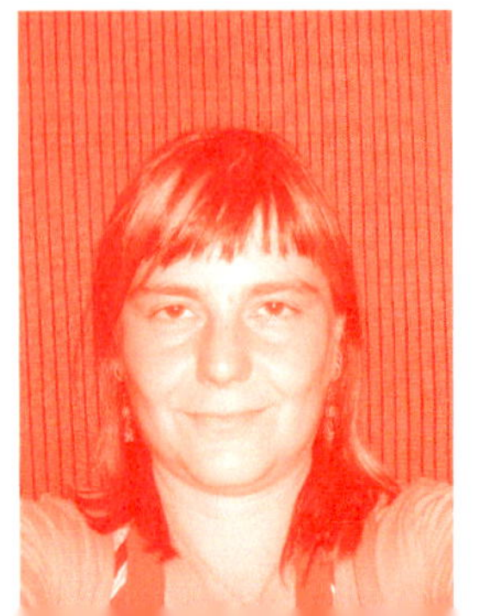
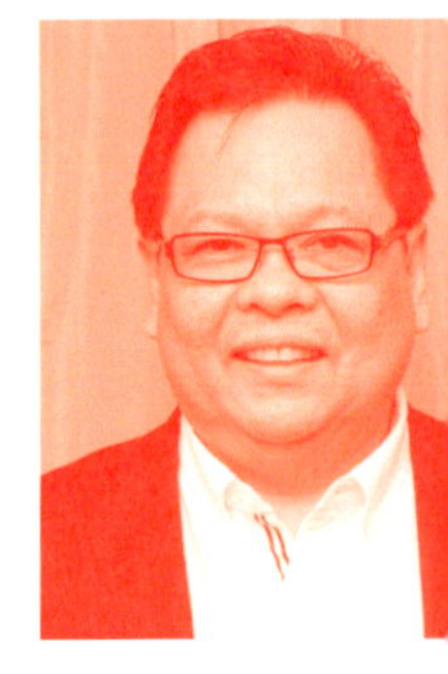
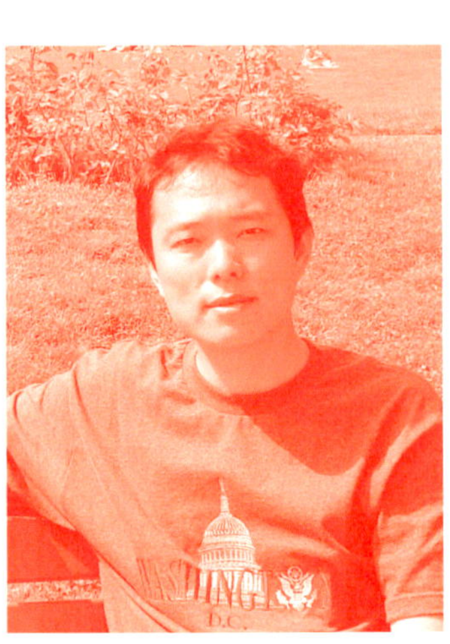

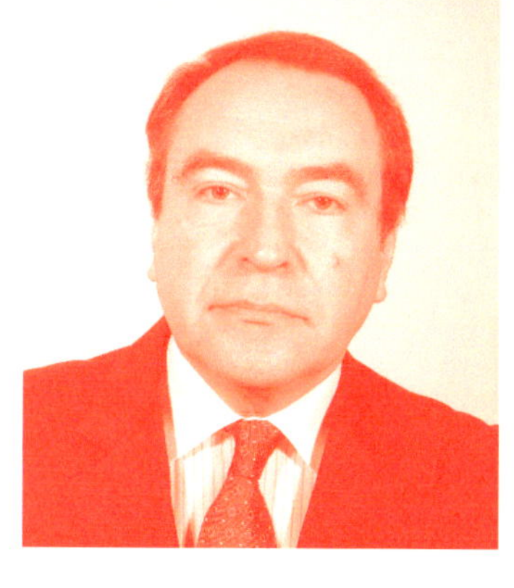

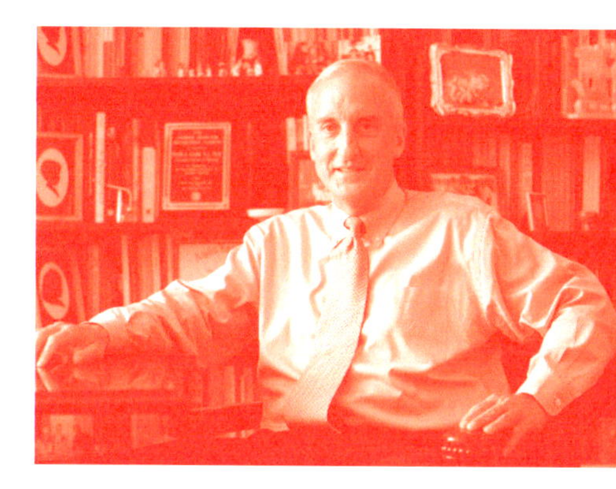

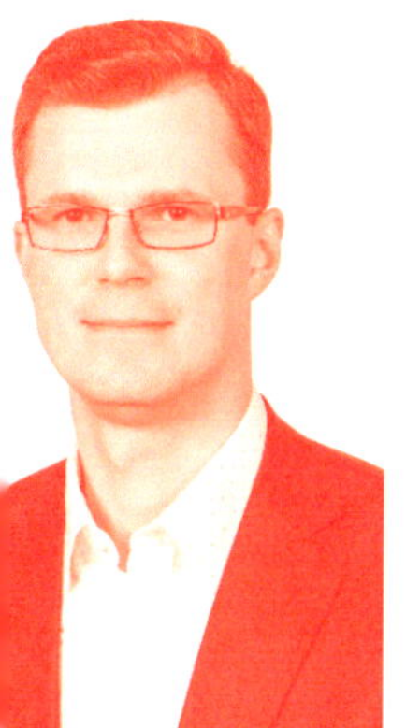

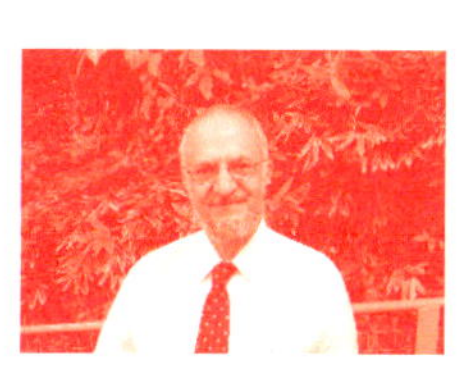

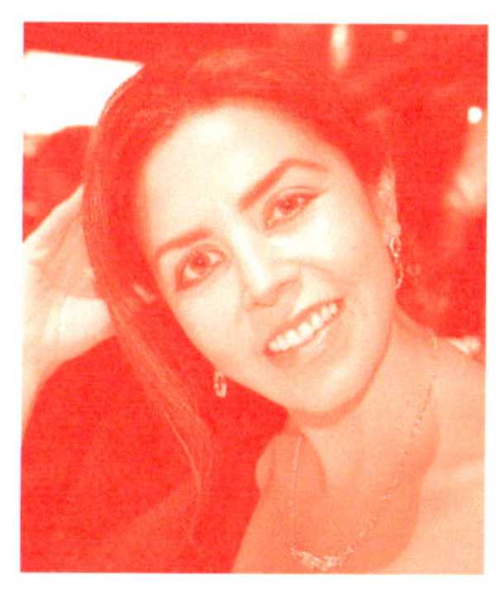

Supporting open minds since 2005

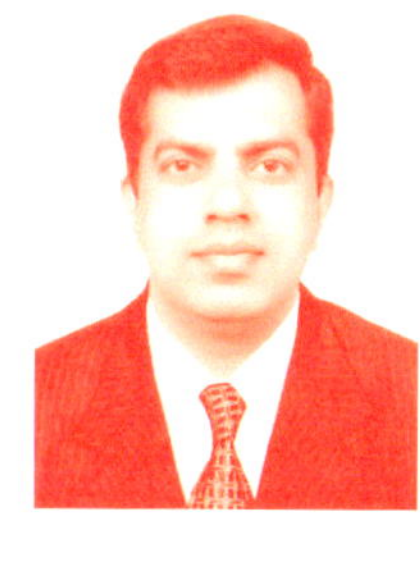

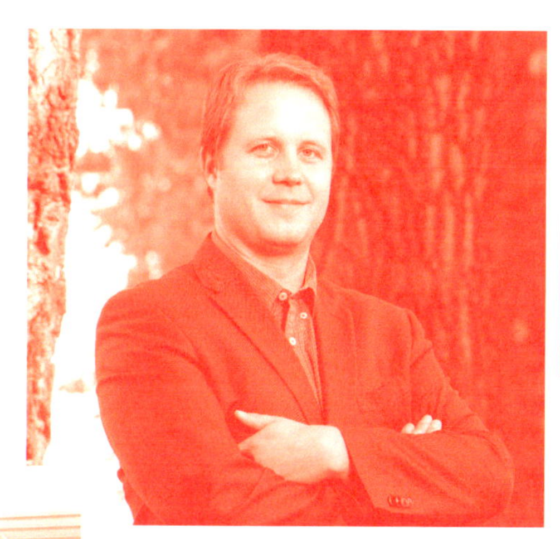

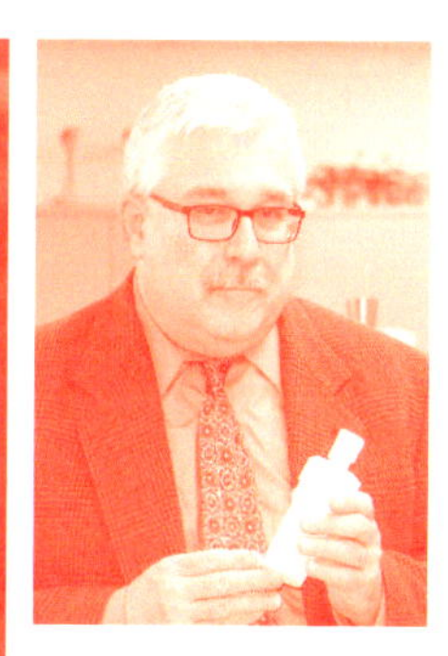

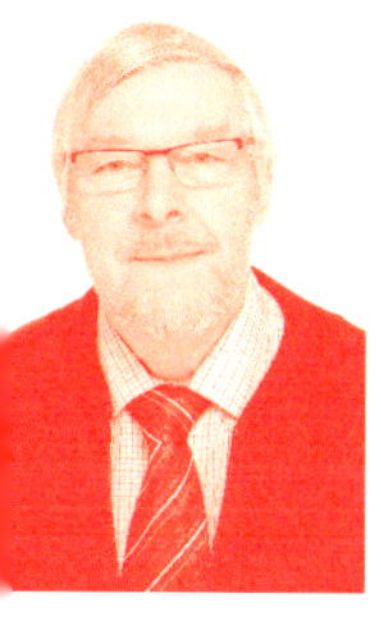

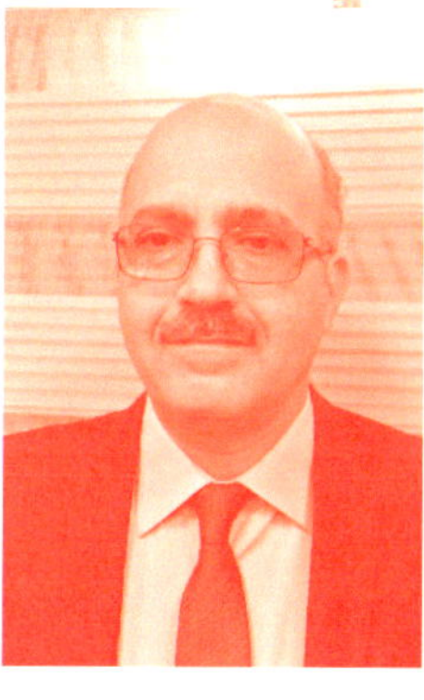

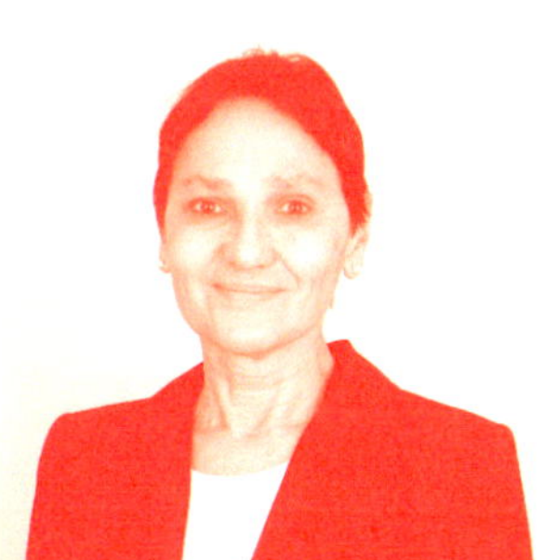

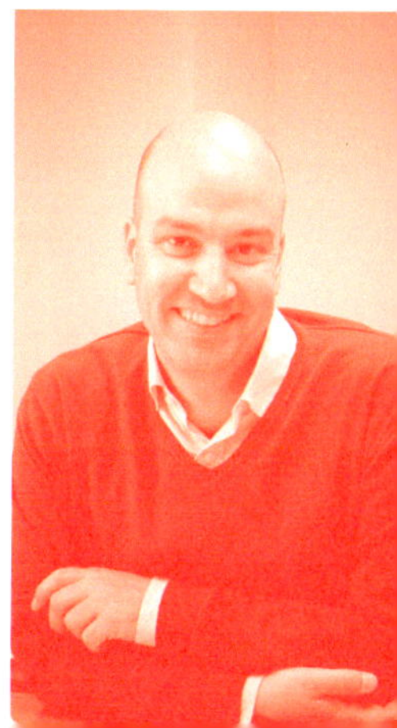

Recent Advances in Gout
http://dx.doi.org/10.5772/intechopen.77945
Edited by Rie Kurose

Part of IntechOpen Book Series: Rheumatology, Volume 4
Book Series Editor: Maria Maślińska

Contributors
Maxim Eliseev, Maria Chikina, Evgeny Nasonov, Pramod Kumar Sharma, Siddhartha Dutta, Dr. Arup Kumar Misra, Rajit Sahai, Narottam Pal, Youming Zhang, Dewen Yan, Rie Kurose

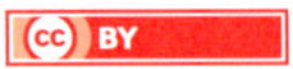

First published in London, United Kingdom, 2020 by IntechOpen
IntechOpen is the global imprint of INTECHOPEN LIMITED, registered in England and Wales, registration number: 11086078, 7th floor, 10 Lower Thames Street, London, EC3R 6AF, United Kingdom
Printed in Croatia

British Library Cataloguing-in-Publication Data
A catalogue record for this book is available from the British Library

Additional hard and PDF copies can be obtained from orders@intechopen.com

Recent Advances in Gout
Edited by Rie Kurose
p. cm.
Print ISBN 978-1-78984-321-7
Online ISBN 978-1-78984-322-4
eBook (PDF) ISBN 978-1-83880-119-9
ISSN 2631-9233

For EU product safety concerns:
IN TECH d.o.o., Prolaz Marije Krucifikse Kozulić 3, 51000 Rijeka, Croatia, info@intechopen.com or visit our website at intechopen.com.

IntechOpen Book Series

Rheumatology

Volume 4

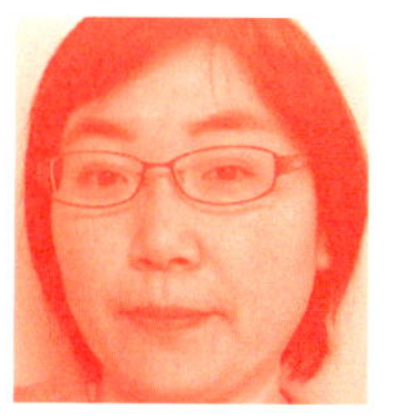

Rie Kurose is a rheumatologist and orthopedic surgeon with extensive experience and management skills. She works for Hirosaki Memorial Hospital, Hirosaki, Japan. She acquired her M.D. and Ph.D. after graduating from Niigata University, Niigata, Japan. As a rheumatologist, she has received the honorable award of annual scientific meeting in American College of Rheumatology and is responsible for the Council of the Japan College of Rheumatology. Currently, she has obtained the Grants-in-Aid for Scientific Research in Japan, and mainly studies basic research on rheumatology.

Editor of Volume 4:
Rie Kurose
Department of Orthopedic Surgery
Hirosaki Memorial Hospital, Hirosaki, Japan

Book Series Editor:
Maria Maślińska
National Institute of Geriatrics, Rheumatology and Rehabilitation
Early Arthritis Clinic, Warsaw, Poland

Scope of the Series

This book series presents new concepts of pathogenesis, including genetic, epigenetic determinants and epidemiology of rheumatic diseases. It focuses on current classification criteria, recommendations for the diagnosis and treatment of rheumatic diseases. The goal of the series is to explain various aspects of disorders associated with impaired immune response and autoimmunity processes. It also discusses risk factors associated with the development of autoimmune diseases, as well as latest discoveries and future perspectives of this extremely dynamic field of internal medicine - rheumatology.

Contents

Preface

Gout is a disease that has a long history and has been known since before the Common Era.

When the uric acid level in blood rises and hyperuricemia persists for a while, urate crystals precipitate in the joints. When these crystals are processed by leukocytes, a gout attack occurs. If the hyperuricemia continues, lifestyle-related diseases such as obesity, arteriosclerosis, and hypertension often develop. Therefore, it is important to treat gouty arthritis, control hyperuricemia, and manage the complications to improve the lifestyle.

This book is a compilation of chapters describing gout, management, ongoing research, and new strategies for treating gout. All of these chapters are authoritative and accomplished discussions that provide novel perspectives on gout topics.

Rie Kurose
Department of Orthopedic Surgery,
Hirosaki Memorial Hospital,
Hirosaki, Japan

Chapter 1

Introductory Chapter: Gout

Rie Kurose

1. Introduction

Gout is a disease known since before the Common Era. There are reports of urate crystal deposition in the big toe joints of an excavated mummy in ancient Egypt. There are records of many figures throughout Western history who experienced the painful suffering of gout, for example, Alexander the Great of Macedonia, King Carlos V of Spain, Frederick the Great of Prussia, Louis XIV of France, Martin Luther of the Reformation, Oliver Cromwell of the Puritan Revolution, the artist Michelangelo, Leonardo da Vinci, the poets Dante and Milton, the physicist Isaac Newton, and the biologist Charles Darwin, among others. In contrast, there is little historical evidence of gout in Asia. Yet the disease has become common in modern society [1–3]. The prevalence of gout in the past has generally been higher among middle-aged men, but in recent years, the number of young people and women with gout has been increasing.

2. Pathophysiology

Gout is a metabolic disorder caused by hyperuricemia [4, 5]. Uric acid is the final metabolite of purine in humans. Uric acid is produced via hypoxanthine and xanthine by the action of xanthine oxidase on purine. Two thirds of uric acid is excreted in the urine and one-third in feces. The amount of serum uric acid is determined by the amount produced and the amount excreted in the kidneys. Hyperuricemia occurs when the level of serum uric acid rises. In hyperuricemia, when urate crystals precipitate in the joint cavity and are phagocytosed by leukocytes, crystal-induced gouty arthritis develops. The symptoms of crystal-induced arthritis are similar to those of rheumatoid arthritis, infectious arthritis, and many collagen diseases, among others. Therefore, it is necessary to distinguish among these conditions. Gouty arthritis develops as acute monoarthritis, with pain, swelling, redness, and fever, peaking in 12–24 h. The initial strong inflammation improves in about 2 weeks but can relapse if hyperuricemia remains unchecked. If hyperuricemia continues, urate crystals are deposited in the joints and connective tissues, activating monocytes or macrophages via the Toll-like receptor pathway and innate immune response. Inflammatory cytokines including interleukin-1β (IL-1β) and tumor necrosis factor-α (TNF-α) are secreted, leading to endothelial activation and attraction of neutrophils to the site of inflammation. Neutrophils secrete inflammatory mediators that create an acidic environment, which causes further precipitation of urate crystals.

3. Classification

Causes of hyperuricemia are classified into primary and secondary hyperuricemia. Primary hyperuricemia is idiopathic. Secondary hyperuricemia can involve

IntechOpen

hereditary metabolic diseases such as Lesch–Nyhan syndrome, phosphoribosyl-pyrophosphate synthetase hypertrophy and congenital myogenic hyperuricemia, malignant tumors such as malignant lymphoma and breast cancer, psoriasis vulgaris, hemolytic anemia, rhabdomyolysis, hypothyroidism, and others. In addition, drug-induced hyperuricemia owing to anticancer agents, low-dose aspirin, loop diuretics, ethambutol, theophylline, and others can be involved in secondary hyperuricemia [6, 7].

4. Symptoms

In gouty arthritis, severe pain attacks may also occur in the hallux metatarso-phalangeal joints, ankle joints, Achilles tendon, knee joints, wrist joints, and other sites [8]. When urate crystals precipitate in the joints, acute inflammatory arthritis is produced, which causes recurrent episodes of red, tender, swollen joints and leads to bone and joint destruction. Gout nodules, or tophi, are most often found in the auricle but also form on the elbow, forearm, hallux, Achilles tendon, patella, and so on. Tophi are not painful, but if they progress, tophi can lead to joint deformation and bone destruction, seriously affecting quality of life. Urate crystal accumulation in the kidneys causes severe pain and deterioration of kidney function and renal failure. Furthermore, hyperuricemia might be associated with hypertension and ischemic heart diseases [9].

5. Management

For effective treatment of acute gout attacks, nonsteroidal anti-inflammatory drugs (NSAIDs) or colchicine are administered as soon as possible, as first-line treatment options [10]. For patients who do not respond to NSAIDs or colchicine, systemic corticosteroids generally may be applied. In addition, for gouty arthritis, joint injection of corticosteroids is often used. For the treatment of chronic gout, drugs are used that either promote uric acid excretion, such as probenecid, or prevent its synthesis via inhibition of enzyme xanthine oxidase, such as allopurinol and febuxostat. If serum uric acid levels fluctuate during gout treatment, arthritis may become exacerbated. In addition, if a gout attack occurs during drug treatment, the level of serum uric acid should be maintained, that is, the amount of uric acid-lowering drugs should not be increased. In such cases, NSAIDs, colchicine, and corticosteroids are used for treatment of a gout attack. Generally, renal function should be checked before drug treatment because gout often occurs in patients with renal impairment. Furthermore, as nondrug treatment, extracorporeal shock wave lithotripsy is used to break up kidney and ureteral stones. Large gout nodules may be surgically resected. Thus, other treatments for gout are often used in combination with drug therapy.

6. New treatment

Gout is classified within a group of autoinflammatory diseases that includes hereditary periodic fever, Muckle-Wells syndrome, familial Mediterranean fever, familial cold autoinflammatory syndrome, and pseudogout. In gout, innate immunity is said to act, and acquired immunity is not involved; there is a difference between gout and autoimmune diseases such as rheumatoid arthritis or juvenile idiopathic arthritis. Recently, newer treatment options have been extensively studied, especially IL-1 inhibitors such as anakinra, canakimumab, and rilonacept. Although IL-1 inhibitors are less effective than TNF inhibitors in rheumatoid arthritis, they have become available as a treatment for gout in recent years. Although the inflammatory effects of IL-1 are diverse, owing to their therapeutic effect, IL-1 inhibitors are expected to be widely used in future clinical applications [11]. When combined with current traditional therapies, these new agents present more promising treatment options for clinicians and patients with gout that is difficult to treat.

7. Conclusion

Gout is not a life-threatening illness, but it is characterized by many lifestyle-related diseases such as obesity, hyperlipidemia, hypertension, and glucose intolerance [12]. All these diseases cause arteriosclerosis; therefore, it is necessary to treat gout carefully. All physicians in clinical practice should know about the treatment and prevention of gout. The treatment goal for gout is to provide effective methods of treatment and prevention and to provide patients with good health-related quality of life. However, long time is required to improve serum uric acid levels and to manage gout attacks. In this book, each expert reports on gout based on the evidence and their own research. It is my hope that this book will be helpful in your clinical practice.

Author details

Rie Kurose
Department of Orthopedic Surgery, Hirosaki Memorial Hospital, Hirosaki, Japan

*Address all correspondence to: riekuro@hirosaki-kinen.or.jp

References

[1] Ogura T, Matsuura K, Matsumoto Y, Mimura Y, Kishida M, Otsuka F, et al. Recent trends of hyperuricemia and obesity in Japanese male adolescents 1991 through 2002. Metabolism. 2004;**53**:448-453

[2] Arromdee E, Michet CJ, Crowson CS, O'Fallon WM, Gabriel SE. Epidemiology of gout: Is the incidence rising? The Journal of Rheumatology. 2002;**29**:2403-2406

[3] Chen SY, Chen CL, Shen ML, Kamatani N. Trends in the manifestations of gout in Taiwan. Rheumatology. 2003;**42**:1529-1533

[4] Campion EW, Glynn RJ, DeLabry LO. Asymptomatic hyperuricemia. Risks and consequences in the normative aging study. The American Journal of Medicine. 1987;**82**:421-426

[5] Shoji A, Yamanaka H, Kamatani N. A retrospective study of the relationship between serum urate level and recurrent attacks of gouty arthritis: Evidence for reduction of recurrent gouty arthritis with antihyperuricemic therapy. Arthritis & Rheumatology. 2004;**51**:321-325

[6] Yamamoto T, Moriwaki Y, Suda M, Takahashi S, Hiroishi K, Higashino K. Theophylline-induced increase in plasma uric acid—Purine catabolism increased by theophylline. International Journal of Clinical Pharmacology Therapy and Toxicology. 1991;**29**:257-261

[7] Erickson AR, Enzenauer RJ, Nordstrom DM, Merenich JA. The prevalence of hypothyroidism in gout. The American Journal of Medicine. 1994;**97**:231-234

[8] Rigby AS, Wood PH. Serum uric acid levels and gout: What does this herald for the population? Clinical and Experimental Rheumatology. 1994;**12**:395-400

[9] Mellen PB, Bleyer AJ, Erlinger TP, Evans GW, Nieto FJ, Wagenknecht LE, et al. Serum uric acid predicts incident hypertension in a biethnic cohort: The atherosclerosis risk in communities study. Hypertension. 2006;**48**:1037-1042

[10] Zhang W, Doherty M, Bardin T, Pascual E, Barskova V, Conaghan P, et al. EULAR Standing Committee for International Clinical Studies Including Therapeutics. EULAR evidence based recommendations for gout. Part II: Management. Report of a task force of the EULAR Standing Committee for International Clinical Studies Including Therapeutics (ESCISIT). Annals of the Rheumatic Diseases. 2006;**65**(10):1312-1324

[11] So A, Dumusc A, Nasi S. The role of IL-1 in gout: From bench to bedside. Rheumatology. 2018;**57**:i12-i19

[12] Zhang T, Pope JE. Cardiovascular effects of urate-lowering therapies in patients with chronic gout: A systematic review and meta-analysis. Rheumatology. 2017;**56**(7):1144-1153

Chapter 2

The Gout

Narottam Pal

Abstract

Gout is a form of arthritis in an individual accompanied with symptoms like severe pain, stiffness, and swelling of one or more joints. Factors that influence rates of gout are many like drinking alcohol, being overweight, drinking soda, becoming dehydrated, the weather, poorly fitting shoes, medical treatments, and many more. The root cause of this condition mainly we can say is the disorder of purine metabolism. There are diagnostic options like synovial fluid test, blood test for uric acid, and differential diagnosis. Preventive measures can include both lifestyle changes and medications. In a recent trend, many treatment options are available like the use of NSAIDs, colchicine, steroids, etc. Common drugs which are on use are probenecid, allopurinol, febuxostat, and pegloticase. Our medical fraternity and researchers are continuing to work on further development.

Keywords: gout, arthritis, purine, uric acid, metabolism

1. Introduction

Gout is a disease condition which often is considered as a form of inflammatory arthritis [1–4]. Unlike arthritis, gout is not a degenerative process. It's generally characterized by frequent attacks of swelling [5, 6], redness, and a tender, warm, and puffy expression of bone joint areas. **Figures 1–3** represent a few gouty expressions. The joints of limbs especially lower limbs, at the base part of the big toe and at the first joint of forefingers of upper limbs, are affected. Some other complications associated are like tophus, urate nephropathy, or kidney stones.

Gout is the result of persistently increased levels of uric acid in the blood [7]. An enzyme named xanthine oxidase is mainly responsible for the production of uric acid in our body. **Figure 4** explains the synthesis pathway of uric acid. As the uric acid concentration becomes high, it undergoes crystallization, and the crystals get deposited in joints. Thus, the surrounding tissues get affected which may lead to redness, swelling, and inflammation, resulting in an attack of gout.

2. Cause

Gout is a result of a disorder in purine metabolism. When there is an increase in the uric acid level in blood, there is a chance of crystallization of uric acid. Such crystals are deposited in joints which start showing the symptoms of gout. The predominant reason of increased level of blood urea is the reduced amount of excretion of uric acid from the body. Synthesis of excessive amount of uric acid may be another reason for increased level in blood, but the cases are more where the first reason is predominant. The risk of developing the symptoms is more

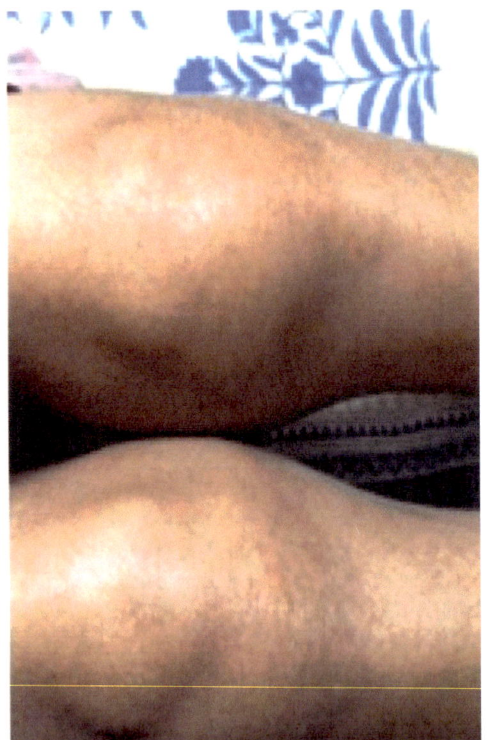

Figure 1.
Swelling in the knee.

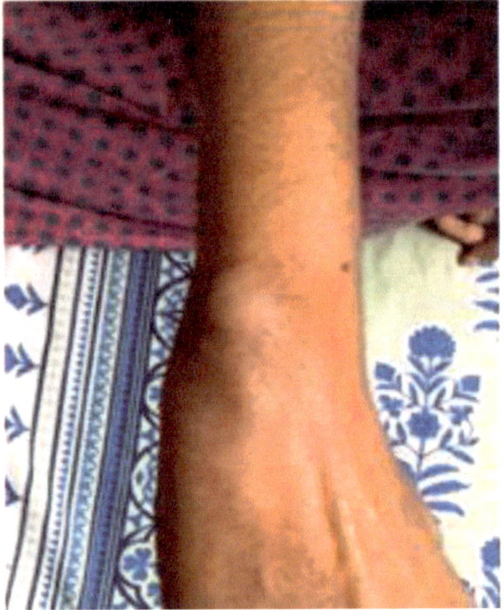

Figure 2.
Puffy wrist (ulna).

and faster as the concentration of uric acid increases. The normal uric acid level in the human body is 2.4–6.0 mg/dL in the case of female and 3.4–7.0 mg/dL in the case of male. When levels are between approximately 7 and 8.9 mg/dL, the

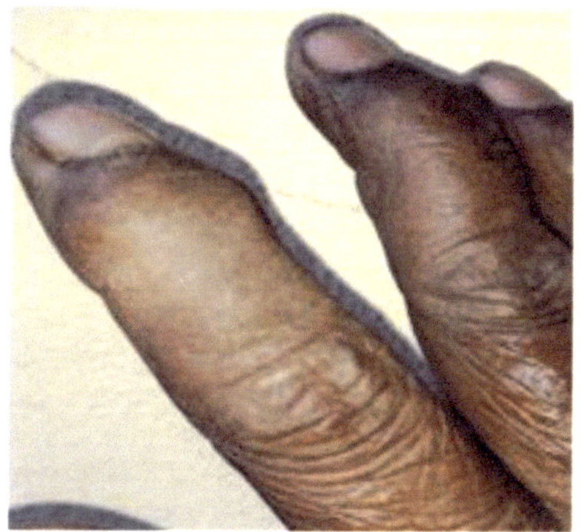

Figure 3.
Swelling and stiff finger.

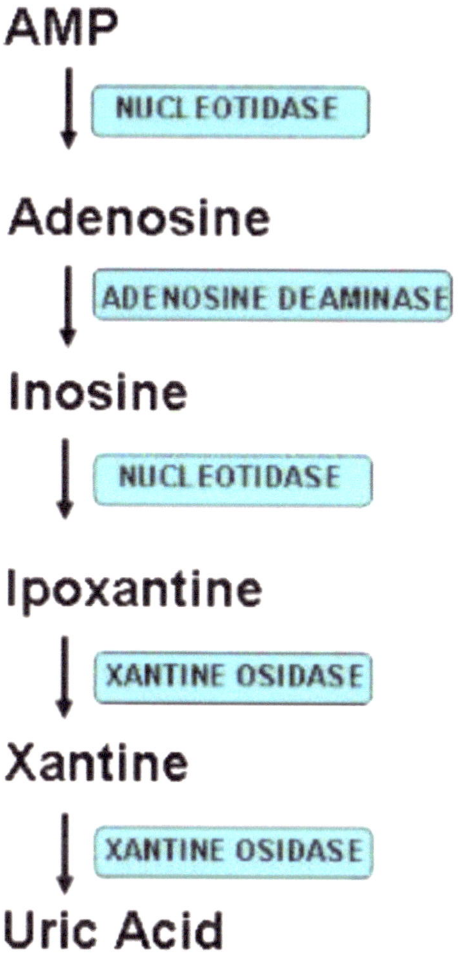

Figure 4.
Part of uric acid pathway.

approximate risk is 0.5% per year. The risk may extend up to 4.5% in those with a level more than 9 mg/dL [8].

Uric acid, when it is in higher level in blood, crystallizes in the form of a salt, monosodium urate, precipitating and making deposition in joints, on tendons, and also in the surrounding tissues. These deposits may be walled off by the ring of certain proteins, which can block the interaction of these crystals with cells and therefore can avoid inflammation. Crystals may break and be displaced out due to the minor physical stress-related damage to the joint like medical or surgical stress or otherwise rapid changes in uric acid levels or so. When they disintegrate through the tophi, they stimulate a local immune-mediated physical-chemical inflammatory reaction in macrophages. This is initiated by an inflammation-mediating protein complex named NLRP3. In the mechanism of inflammation, a protein named interleukin 1β plays an important role which is obtained from pro-interleukin 1β with the help of enzyme caspase 1. NLRP3 assists the enzyme in its function.

3. Diagnosis

Sign and symptoms of arthritis may motivate the physician to go for examination of the patient. It can be diagnosed by different investigational methods. Patients with hyperuricemia can receive treatment based on the diagnosis and their severity. Different types of diagnosis are mentioned as follows.

3.1 Blood tests

Since hyperuricemia is a cause for uric acid crystallization and deposition of the same on joints, examination of blood sample is a common and initial process observed in orthopedic clinics [9, 10]. But sometimes it's observed that gout occurs without hyperuricemia also and many people with increased uric acid levels did not develop gout. Thus, the usefulness of the diagnosis of measuring uric acid levels in many individuals is limited. The normal uric acid level in blood is ranging around or less than 420 μmol/L (7.0 mg/dL) in males and 360 μmol/L (6.0 mg/dL) in females. Therefore, above this margin of uric acid in blood may be considered as hyperuricemia. Other blood sample investigations commonly performed are erythrocyte sedimentation rate (ESR), white blood cell count, kidney function and electrolyte tests.

3.2 Synovial fluid

A qualitative investigation of gout is based upon polarimetric analysis of crystals of monosodium urate [11]. These crystals are deposited on the joints of a hyperuricemic patient. A synovial fluid sample is collected from undiagnosed inflamed joints with the help of arthrocentesis. The fluid is sampled appropriately to examine these crystals. In a polarimeter the sample is studied to check the needle-like morphology as well as strong negative birefringence.

3.3 Miscellaneous methods

There are certain investigations which may or may not be directly related to arthritis but definitely prove beneficial most of the time [12]. Detection for psoriatic arthritis is one of them. Since it can affect joints on either one side or both sides of our body, the signs and symptoms of this often resemble those of arthritis. The disease causes joints to become painful, swollen, puffy, and warm to the touch. Another important test is for septic arthritis. This may be accompanied by joint infection. Naturally the disease results in joint inflammation. Other symptoms typically include heat, redness, and pain in a single joint which may be associated with a decreased ability in moving the joint. One more diagnosis may be recommended, and that is to test for reactive arthritis. This can affect the heels, fingers, toes, low back portion, and joints, especially of the ankles and knees [13, 14].

4. Preventive measures

In mild to moderate cases of gout, lifestyle changes can decrease uric acid levels in blood. These modifications may include selection of correct diet, regular and appropriate exercise, and consultation with a physician. Physiotherapy also can help in this regard.

4.1 Food habit

Appropriate diet is very important [15]. Overweight is a big factor causing joint pain [16]. Food containing high amounts of purine such as seafood like shellfish, anchovies, sardines, herring, codfish, mussels, scallops, trout haddock, etc.; some meats, such as turkey, bacon, veal, venison, and organ meats like liver, etc. [17]; and drinks and beverages like beer or all types of alcoholic beverages, containing high amounts of purine, can increase blood urea level [18]. Soft drink contains either fructose or sucrose in huge quantity which may enhance the precipitation of uric acid crystals. Therefore, reducing or omitting such products from the diet list is advisable.

4.2 Sleep apnea

As there is a chance of deficiency of oxygen in the cell due to improper breathing or irregular breathing style during sleep, it may stimulate the release of purine from those cells, and therefore a control on sleep apnea may help in the control of gout.

4.3 Dehydration

Becoming dehydrated may also be a reason of gout risk. Exact mechanism is not clear, but it is believed that it may increase the concentration of uric acid in reduced volume of blood and also in the joint fluid. Hence, consuming adequate amount of water is advisable.

4.4 Obesity

Obesity, diabetes, and increased cholesterol are conditions quite commonly seen together. If these two disorders become contemporary in a patient, he or she may land up with a metabolic syndrome. Such patients frequently also have an elevated level of uric acid in their blood. In certain time diuretics prescribed to control high blood pressure also can cause higher levels of uric acid.

4.5 Drinking soda

Carbonated water for drinks or drinking soda has a high-fructose corn syrup which is a culprit in elevating uric acid levels, thereby increasing gout risk.

4.6 Kidney stones

In a certain time, kidney stone may get traces of uric acid. In such cases if dehydration takes place in the patient's body, then precipitation of uric acid becomes more severe. To prevent dehydration, drinking sufficient amount of water a day is very essential.

4.7 Poorly fitting shoes

Wearing the wrong shoes can become another gout-triggering factor. Any kind of trauma or damage to an area can cause a gout pain and swelling in susceptible people. If our shoes rub the toe or nearby area of our feet, then it can contribute to a gout attack. So it is better to make sure that the toe area of our shoes is wide enough so that it can accommodate our feet without pinching or rubbing.

4.8 Medical treatments

Toxic effect of some drug substances can contribute in hyperuricemia. These drug substances are recommended for patients for certain disease conditions where they are certainly beneficial but may result in elevated uric acid level. Diuretics can decrease the removal of uric acid from our body and cause hyperuricemia, thereby a risk factor to develop gout. In the treatment of carcinoma, chemotherapy may lead to the breakdown and rapid turnover of tissue cells and can lead to increased synthesis of uric acid. In case of surgery, a sudden severe physiological change that causes reduced blood flowing to the area of peripheral joints can also be a risk factor for gout. Therefore, adequate amounts of precautions are required while receiving treatment.

5. Medications

Many drug substances are available for the treatment of hyperuricemia. As a first-line therapy along with these drugs, a compound is to be recommended which can cause a symptomatic relief. One of the best choices is an anti-inflammatory agent.

Available drugs recommended for reducing hyperuricemia are allopurinol, febuxostat, probenecid, pegloticase, lesinurad, etc.

Allopurinol is a structural isomer of hypoxanthine (a naturally existing purine in our body) and acts to inhibit an enzyme xanthine oxidase [19]. In the presence of this enzyme, allopurinol will be converted to a compound named alloxanthine, and thereby the formation of uric acid from hypoxanthine and xanthine will be inhibited.

Febuxostat is not a purine-based compound but a selective inhibitor of enzyme xanthine oxidase [20–24]. In contrast to allopurinol, this compound inhibits both oxidized and reduced forms of enzyme xanthine oxidase and has minimal effects on other enzymes of pyrimidine and purine metabolism. A study comparing febuxostat to allopurinol revealed that more individuals receiving febuxostat had a decreased uric acid level.

Therapeutically, probenecid is generally coadministered with other pharmacologically active substances such as anti-inflammatory drugs or penicillins resulting in a substantial diminished renal clearance of all these compounds [25–28]. In higher doses than are actually required for the uricosuric effect, probenecid can inhibit the transport system which removes acid substances from the cerebrospinal fluid. Probenecid also increases the urinary excretion of uric acid and therefore has a therapeutic value for the ailment of gout.

Pegloticase is a third-line treatment option for those in whom other treatment options are not tolerated [29]. Generally it is an option for the treatment of chronic, severe, treatment-refractory gout. Pegloticase, a PEGylated, recombinant uricase enzyme, converts salt of uric acid into allantoin. Thus, it makes a wonderful job by increasing the excretion of uric acid through kidney filtration.

Lesinurad is a drug of choice to be recommended together with either febuxostat or allopurinol when these medications are not sufficient as monotherapy [30, 31]. It reduces urate transport by inhibiting a protein named URAT1 that is responsible for much reabsorption of uric acid or urat in the kidneys. It also inhibits the OAT4 protein, which is associated with hyperuricemic condition caused by diuretic drugs.

A confirmation about a gout case is given by medical experts only after certain tests are conducted and analyzed. Prior to the investigation, a physician can go for a symptomatic relief for the suffering patients by providing a simple prescription containing simple anti-inflammatory or analgesic drugs (NSAIDs) [32, 33]. Common compounds are like acetaminophen, ibuprofen, indomethacin, ketorolac, piroxicam, mefenamic acid, etc. A selective COX-2 inhibitor can be a better choice in case a physician looks for the therapy for beyond 1 week. These drugs include meloxicam, celecoxib, rofecoxib, etoricoxib, etc. All the abovementioned drugs come under nonsteroidal anti-inflammatory drugs. With similar efficacy corticosteroidal drugs also are also recommended as a co-prescription for symptomatic control. Both glucocorticoids and mineralocorticoids can be prescribed depending on the case demand. Some examples of synthetic corticosteroids are betamethasone, prednisone, prednisolone, triamcinolone, methylprednisolone, dexamethasone, and systemic (oral and injectable) steroids that are available for use including hydrocortisone, cortisone ethamethasoneb, fludrocortisone, etc. For those patients unable to tolerate NSAIDs, colchicine is an ideal alternative. Colchicine is a category of substance which is effective at lower dose, and it is well tolerated [34]. It may interact with some other commonly prescribed drug substances, such as erythromycin and atorvastatin, simvastatin, etc.

6. Conclusion

Gout is a form of disease which may be acute or chronic, associated with symptoms like severe pain, stiffness, and swelling of one or more joints. It occurs due to increased production of uric acid in our body or reduced excretion of the same from our body. Such metabolic disorder may arise from poor lifestyle and improper food habits. A number of diagnostic options are available and treatment too. But it's always advisable to adapt a healthy food habit, practice physical exercise, and continue with physician's consultation and medication to get rid of this disease condition.

Acknowledgements

We are very much thankful to Dr. A. Srinivasa Rao, principal and professor, Bhaskar Pharmacy College, Hyderabad, for his guidance, kind help, and constant encouragement during the progress of this chapter writing work. We also express our gratitude to Dr. V.V. Rao, CEO, and Mr. J.V. Krishna Rao, secretary, JB Group of Educational Institution, for providing a healthy professional environment which is an essence in any profession. We express heartful thanks to Dr. Ratnakar Rao K, senior consultant orthopedic surgeon, Continental Hospitals, Hyderabad, India; Dr. B. Sandeep Kumar, resident, Care hospitals, Hyderabad, India; and Dr. S. Shekar Reddy, assistant professor, Bhaskar Medical College, Hyderabad, India, for providing valuable information and providing opportunities to get exposure to patients suffering from the very disease.

Author details

Narottam Pal
Bhaskar Pharmacy College, Hyderabad, India

*Address all correspondence to: narottampal8224@gmail.com

References

[1] Brunton LL, Lgzo JS, Parker KL. Goodman and Gilman's the Pharmacological Basis of Therapeutics. 11th ed. New York: McGraw-Hill; 2006. pp. 706-711

[2] Walker R, Whittlesea C. Clinical Pharmacy and Therapeutics. 5th ed. Churchill Livingstone; 2012. pp. 848-857

[3] Finkel R, Clark MA, Cubeddu LX. Lippincott's Illustrated Reviews: Pharmacology. 5th ed. Vol. 2013. Wolter Kluwer (India Pvt. Ltd.). pp. 515-517

[4] Rang HP, Dale MM, Ritter JM, Flower RJ. Rang and Dale Pharmacology. 6th ed. Churchill Livingstone; 2008. pp. 238-239

[5] Chen LX, Schumacher HR. Gout: An evidence-based review. Journal of Clinical Rheumatology. 2008;**14**(5 Suppl):S55-S62. DOI: 10.1097/RHU.0b013e3181896921

[6] Beyl RN Jr, Hughes L, Morgan S. Update on importance of diet in gout. The American Journal of Medicine. 2016;**129**(11):1153-1158. DOI: 10.1016/j.amjmed.2016.06.040. PMID 27452679

[7] Richette P, Bardin T. Gout. Lancet. 2010;**375**(9711):318-328. DOI: 10.1016/S0140-6736(09)60883-7

[8] Terkeltaub R. Update on gout: New therapeutic strategies and options. Nature Reviews Rheumatology. 2010;**6**(1):30-38. DOI: 10.1038/nrrheum.2009.236

[9] Sachs L, Batra KL, Zimmermann B. Medical implications of hyperuricemia. Medicine and Health, Rhode Island. 2009;**92**(11):353-355

[10] Gout: Differential Diagnoses & Workup—eMedicine Rheumatology. Medscape. Archived from the original on 2010-07-25

[11] Sturrock R. Gout. Easy to misdiagnose. BMJ. 2000;**320**(7228):132-133. DOI: 10.1136/bmj.320.7228.132

[12] Firestein GS, Budd RC, Harris ED Jr, McInnes IB, Ruddy S, Sergent JS, Chapter 87: Gout and hyperuricemia. Kelley's Textbook of Rheumatology (8th ed.). 2008. Elsevier. ISBN 978-1-4160-4842-8

[13] Abrams B. Sleep apnea as a cause of gout flares. The Medscape Journal of Medicine. 2009;**11**(1):3

[14] Dalbeth N, Merriman TR, Stamp LK. Gout. Lancet. 2016;**388**(10055):2039-2052. DOI: 10.1016/s0140-6736(16)00346-9

[15] Rich Man's Disease—definition of Rich Man's Disease in the medical dictionary. Free Online Medical Dictionary, Thesaurus and Encyclopedia

[16] Stein JJ, Cush AK, Michael C. Rheumatology: Diagnosis and Therapeutics. 2nd ed. Philadelphia: Lippincott, Williams & Wilkins; 2005. p. 192. ISBN 9780781757324. Archived from the original on 2017-09-08

[17] Kaneko K, Aoyagi Y, Fukuuchi T, Inazawa K, Yamaoka N. Total purine and purine base content of common foodstuffs for facilitating nutritional therapy for gout and hyperuricemia. Biological and Pharmaceutical Bulletin. 2014;**37**(5):709-721. DOI: 10.1248/bpb.b13-00967. PMID 24553148

[18] Tanya J, Topless RK, Dalbeth N, Merriman TR. Evaluation of the diet wide contribution to serum urate levels: Meta-analysis of population based cohorts. BMJ. 2018:k3951. DOI: 10.1136/bmj.k3951

[19] Australian Rheumatology Association. Available from: www.rheumatology.org.au [Revised February 2016]

[20] Okamoto K, Eger BT, Nishino T, Kondo S, Pai EF. An extremely potent inhibitor of xanthine oxidoreductase: Crystal structure of the enzyme-inhibitor complex and mechanism of inhibition. The Journal of Biological Chemistry. 2003;**278**:1848-1855

[21] Takano Y, Hase-Aoki K, Horiuchi H, Zhao L, Kasahara Y, Kondo S. Selectivity of febuxostat, a novel non-purine inhibitor of xanthine oxidase/ xanthine dehydrogenase. Life Sciences. 2005;**76**:1835-1847

[22] Yamamoto T, Moriwaki Y, Fujimura Y, Takahashi S, Tsutsumi Z, Tsutsui T, et al. Emerging therapies in the long-term management of hyperuricaemia and gout. Internal Medicine Journal. 2007;**37**(4):258-266

[23] Becker MA, Schumacher HR, Wortmann RL. Febuxostat compared with allopurinol in patients with hyperuricemia and gout. The New England Journal of Medicine. 2005;**353**(23):2450-2461

[24] Pal N, Rao AS, Ravikumar P. New method development and validation for the determination of febuxostat in human plasma by liquid chromatography–mass spectrometry. International Journal of Pharmacy and Pharmaceutical Sciences. 2016;**8**(9):61-70

[25] Cunningham RF, Israili ZH, Dayton PG. Clinical Pharmacokinetics. 1981;**6**:135

[26] van Gulpcn C, Brokerhof AW, van der Kay M, Tjaden UR, Maittie H. Journal of Chromatography. 1986;**568**:365

[27] Roos BE, Wickström G, Hartvig P, Nilsson JLG. European Journal of Clinical Pharmacology. 1980;**17**:223

[28] Hartvig P, Fagerlund C, Emanuelsson BM. Journal of Chromatography. 1982;**228**:340

[29] Krystexxa [prescribing information]. Horizon Pharma Rhematology LLC

[30] Zurampic: EPAR—Product Information (PDF). European Medicines Agency. 2017

[31] FDA Professional Drug Information: Zurampic. [Accessed 19 July 2017]

[32] Durme CM, Wechalekar MD, Buchbinder R, Schlesinger N, van der Heijde D, Landewé RB. Non-steroidal anti-inflammatory drugs for acute gout. The Cochrane Database of Systematic Reviews. 2014;**9**(9):CD010120. DOI: 10.1002/14651858.CD010120.pub2

[33] Information for Healthcare Professionals: New Safety Information for Colchicine (marketed as Colcrys). U.S. Food and Drug Administration. Archived from the original on 2009-10-18

[34] Wechalekar MD, Schlesinger N, Buchbinder R, Aletaha D. Colchicine for acute gout. The Cochrane Database of Systematic Reviews. 2014;**8**(8):CD006190. DOI: 10.1002/14651858.CD006190.pub2

Chapter 3

Pharmacology of the Therapeutic Approaches of Gout

Rajit Sahai, Pramod Kumar Sharma, Arup Misra and Siddhartha Dutta

Abstract

Gout is a metabolic disorder characterized by hyperuricemia. Asymptomatic hyperuricemia ought not to be treated until arthritis; renal calculi or tophi become evident. The cornerstone of therapy of acute attack is often nonsteroidal anti-inflammatory drugs (NSAIDs), barring specific situations wherein colchicine and corticosteroids do have a role. Usually NSAIDs with stronger anti-inflammatory action are used in high and quickly repeated doses and have a slower response response as compared to colchicine, they are better tolerated. Colchicine has a unique mechanism action. Intra-articular corticosteroids provide relief in acute attack and are given in patients having inability to tolerate NSAIDs and colchicine. Chronic gout requires treatments with drugs that either promote excretion (e.g., probenecid, lesinurad) or prevent its synthesis through inhibition of enzyme *xanthine oxidase* (allopurinol, febuxostat, etc.). Pegloticase and rasburicase, being a recombinant uricase enzyme, oxidize uric acid to highly soluble allantoin excreted in urine. In spite of these effective treatment modalities, question arises on their safety profile. Newer treatment options are being extensively studied especially interleukin-1 (IL-1) inhibitors but their approval is still pending. The quest for an optimally designed drug with desirable efficacy and acceptable safety profile is still on.

Keywords: gout, hyperuricemia, arthritis, uricosurics, uricase

1. Introduction

Gout is a metabolic disorder characterized by increased deposition of urate crystals in the joints and connective tissue (tophi) and results in episodic acute or chronic arthritis. It also leads to deposition of urate crystals within the renal interstitium or nephrolithiasis [1]. Prevalence of gout has an uneven distribution throughout the globe with a higher prevalence in the Pacific countries. Blacks have been shown to have a decreased incidence/prevalence [2]. Gout affects 3% people of the western population with majority cases seen in middle-aged and elderly men and postmenopausal women [3]. Gout can be either a primary gout which is hereditary or due to genetic anomaly in the genes responsible for excretion of uric acid. Secondary gout is majorly due to acquired causes of hyperuricemia. Deposition of urate crystal occurs when uric acid levels are >6.8 mg/dl.

IntechOpen

2. Causes

Gout can result from either increased production or due to decreased excretion of uric acid from the kidney or both. The causes of hyperuricemia can be listed separately into those for primary and secondary hyperuricemia.

1. Primary hyperuricemia
    a. Increased production of purine
        i. Idiopathic
        ii. Enzyme defects (e.g., Lesch-Nyhan syndrome, glycogen storage diseases)
    b. Decreased renal clearance
        i. Idiopathic
2. Secondary hyperuricemia
    a. Increased catabolism and turnover of purine
        i. Myeloproliferative disorders
        ii. Lymphoproliferative disorders
        iii. Carcinoma and sarcoma
        iv. Chronic hemolytic anemia
        v. Cytotoxic drugs
        vi. Psoriasis
    b. Decreased renal clearance
        i. Intrinsic kidney disease
        ii. Drug induced (thiazides, low dose aspirin, pyrazinamide, loop diuretics, ethambutol, levodopa, ethanol cyclosporine, etc.)
        iii. Hyperlactacidemia (lactic acidosis, alcoholism)
        iv. Hyperketoacidemia (diabetic ketoacidosis, starvation)
        v. Diabetes insipidus
        vi. Bartter syndrome [4]

3. Pathophysiology

Following hyperuricemia, the urate crystals get deposited in the joints and connective tissues and activate monocytes or macrophages via Toll-like receptor

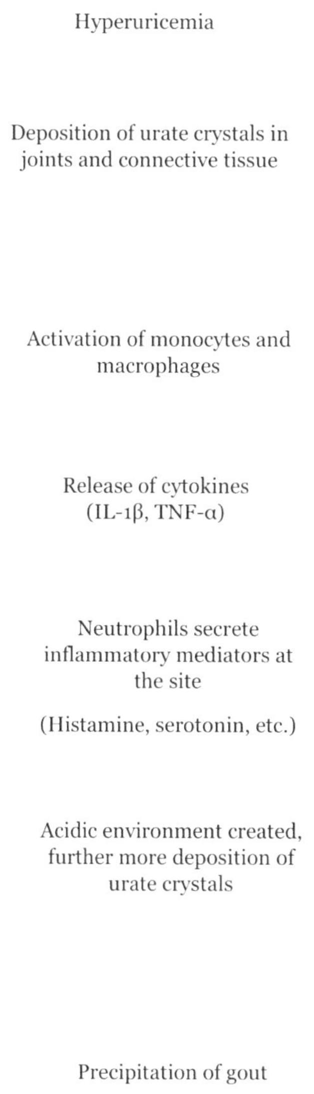

Hyperuricemia

Deposition of urate crystals in joints and connective tissue

Activation of monocytes and macrophages

Release of cytokines (IL-1β, TNF-α)

Neutrophils secrete inflammatory mediators at the site

(Histamine, serotonin, etc.)

Acidic environment created, further more deposition of urate crystals

Precipitation of gout

Figure 1.
Schematic illustration of pathophysiology of gout.

pathway mounting and innate immune response. This results in secretion of cytokines including interleukin-1β (IL-1β) and tumor necrosis factor-α (TNF-α) leading to endothelial activation and attraction of neutrophils to the site of inflammation. Neutrophils secrete inflammatory mediators that create an acidic environment, which further causes precipitation of urate crystals (**Figure 1**) [3].

4. Clinical presentation

Acute arthritis is the commonest early presentation of gout. It usually affects one joint precisely the metatarsophalangeal joint of the great toe. However, the disease can also have a polyarticular presentation and involve other joints like tarsal, ankle, or knee joints. In certain cases, it may also have a periarticular involvement involving the soft tissues. The intensity of the pain increases with the duration of the attack. Joints become swollen, tender with the overlying skin being warm, tense, and red in color. These symptoms most likely are associated with hyperthermia, and with time tophi start developing in the external ears, feet, olecranon, and prepatellar bursa [4, 5].

1. Laboratory investigations:

    a. Serum uric acid levels: Used for diagnosing a patient of gout; however, these could be false positives and false negatives as it may not be raised at the time of the attack. It is also used as a reference while the patient is receiving hypouricemic therapy.

    b. Peripheral leukocyte count is usually elevated during attack.

    c. Aspiration of joint fluid and demonstration of sodium urate crystals are diagnostic. When observed under the microscope, these are needle-shaped crystals present both extracellularly and intracellularly. Increase in the number of crystals within the joint can lead to formation of a thick pasty, chalky joint fluid. When observed under compensated polarized light, the crystals appear to be brightly birefringent with negative elongations. In addition, the leukocyte count of the aspirated fluid is also found to be raised [1, 6].

2. Radiographic imaging:

    a. X-ray: No changes seen in early stage of disease, later punched out erosions with an overhanging rim of cortical bone develop. Presence of this erosion adjacent to tophi is diagnostic.

    b. Ultrasonography: Used when tophi are small and cannot be appreciated physically [4, 5].

5. Management of gout

Treatment modality in gout is aimed at:

1. Reducing the symptoms during acute attack

2. Reducing the recurrent attacks

3. Lowering serum urate levels [3]

Treatment can be divided into non-pharmacological and pharmacological.

5.1 Non-pharmacological treatment

Patients upon being diagnosed with hyperuricemia should be advised diet with less purine content (refined cereals, white bread, milk, peanut butter, fruits, nuts, tomato, green vegetables, etc.). Alcohol consumption should be kept at minimum; intake of whiskey and wine should be preferred rather than beer. Organ meats and beverages sweetened with high fructose corn syrup should be avoided. In addition, high intake of liquid diet should be advised to facilitate urine output of 2 L or more, which favors urate excretion. Patients with asymptomatic hyperuricemia ought not to be given pharmacological treatment until arthritis or renal calculi develop.

5.2 Pharmacological treatment

Pharmacotherapy of gout is divided into:

1. For acute gout

    a. Nonsteroidal anti-inflammatory drugs (NSAIDs)

    b. Colchicine

    c. Corticosteroids

2. For chronic gout

    a. Uricosurics (probenecid, sulfinpyrazone, benzbromarone, lesinurad)

    b. Uric acid synthesis inhibitors (allopurinol, febuxostat)

    c. Uricase (rasburicase, pegloticase) [7]

5.2.1 For acute gout

1. **NSAIDs:** Oral agents are preferred and are effective of acute gout. The drugs with a stronger anti-inflammatory action are used. They provide relief by inhibiting cyclooxygenase-2(COX-2)-mediated prostaglandin synthesis at the site of injury; however, there are certain additional mechanisms pertaining to some drugs also. The NSAIDs provide symptomatic relief from pain and inflammation. In addition, they are also used initially as a bridging therapy along with uric acid synthesis inhibitors to prevent development of symptoms of acute gouty arthritis due to mobilization of urate from the tissues. NSAIDs are contraindicated in conditions like active peptic ulcer disease, impaired kidney function, and history of allergic reactions. The drugs used more often are naproxen, piroxicam, diclofenac, indomethacin, and etoricoxib [5, 8].

    a. **Naproxen:** It is a nonselective COX inhibitor having a stronger anti-inflammatory activity and potent in inhibiting leucocyte migration. Peak anti-inflammatory effect starts after 2–4 weeks.

        i. Pharmacokinetics: It is absorbed in fullest extent after oral administration and is absorbed slowly via rectal route. It is 99% plasma protein bound with a variable $t_{1/2}$. With advancement of age, the renal function declines, and the $t_{1/2}$ increases. It is 30% metabolized in liver, and its excretion occurs via urine. It crosses placenta and is also excreted in milk.

        ii. Dosage: It is started in a dosage of 750 mg stat followed by 250 mg twice or thrice daily.

        iii. Adverse effects: These are mostly gastrointestinal in nature like heartburn, nausea, dyspepsia, abdominal pain, constipation, diarrhea, and stomatitis. CNS side effects like headache, drowsiness, headache, dizziness, and vertigo and other adverse effects like pruritis, diaphoresis, loss of renal function, angioedema, and thrombocytopenia can also occur. Reports also suggest that it can also increase the risk of myocardial infarction [8].

b. **Piroxicam**: Another nonselective COX inhibitor having a potent anti-inflammatory action and longer duration of action. In addition to inhibition of COX enzyme, it has also been proposed to inhibit neutrophil activation and inhibition of proteoglycanase and collagenase in cartilage.

   i. Pharmacokinetics: Completely absorbed upon oral administration and undergoes enterohepatic circulation. It is 99% protein bound and is metabolized in the liver by CYP2C9. t1/2 is approximately between 15 and 20 hours. Steady state plasma concentrations are attained in 7–12 days and further excreted in urine and feces.

   ii. Dosage: It is given in a dose of 20 mg daily.

   iii. Adverse effects: Experienced by 20% of the patients and eventually 5% of the recipients discontinue the treatment. The adverse effects are similar to those of naproxen though more in intensity. It is not a first-line agent for treatment of pain and inflammation in gout among all NSAIDs [9].

c. **Indomethacin**: A potent nonselective COX inhibitor. It also inhibits motility of polymorphonuclear lymphocytes, inhibits synthesis of mucopolysaccharides, and has a direct COX-independent vasoconstrictor effect.

   i. Pharmacokinetics: It has a good bioavailability after oral administration. Peak plasma concentrations are achieved within 1–2 hours. It is 99% plasma protein bound, and concentration within the synovial fluid equals that of plasma concentration in 5 hours of oral administration. It also undergoes enterohepatic circulation due to which it has a variable t1/2 and averages out to be about 2 hours.

   ii. Dosage: It is given in a dose of 25 mg twice of thrice daily or 75–100 mg at night.

   iii. Adverse effects: Experienced by majority of patients but in particular elderly. The gastrointestinal adverse effects are similar as that of naproxen though it can also cause ulcerations within the bowel. Certain CNS adverse effects like headache, dizziness, vertigo, and mental confusion can also occur. It should be prescribed cautiously to patients with epilepsy, psychiatric disorders or Parkinson's disease as they are at more risk of eliciting serious CNS side effects. It can also cause certain hematopoietic disorders like neutropenia, thrombocytopenia, and rarely aplastic anemia. Probenecid increases the plasma concentration of indomethacin, so the dose should be lowered in such case [10].

d. **Etoricoxib**: It is a newer selective COX-2 inhibitor having the highest COX-2-selective activity. It is given only in patients with high risk of peptic ulcer, perforation, or bleeding.

i. Pharmacokinetics: It is incompletely absorbed, has a longer t1/2 between 20 and 60 hours, metabolized in the liver, and excreted via urine. Hepatic impairment promotes its accumulation in the body, whereas renal impairment does not.

ii. Dosage: It is given in a dosage of 60–120 mg once daily.

iii. Adverse effects: Dyspepsia, abdominal pain, pedal edema, rise in BP, dry mouth, aphthous ulcers, taste disturbance, and paresthesias. It should not be used in patients with or at risk of cardiovascular or cerebrovascular disease as it can cause prothrombotic events [9].

2. **Colchicine**: It is one of the oldest drugs available for treatment of acute gout. An alkaloid obtained from *Colchicum autumnale* having no analgesic or anti-inflammatory property nor having any effect on inhibiting synthesis or increasing excretion of uric acid. It is not used as a first-line drug due to its narrow therapeutic window and increased side effects. It suppress gouty inflammation by various mechanisms: It (a) prevents granulocyte migration into the inflamed joint, (b) inhibits release of glycoprotein which causes aggravates inflammation by forming lactic acid and by releasing lysosomal enzymes which lead to joint destruction, and (c) binds to an intracellular protein called tubulin and causes depolymerization and disappearance of microtubules in granulocytes. Collectively, these prevent migration of granulocytes into the area of inflammation and further prevent it. It also limits monosodium urate crystal-induced NALP3 inflammasome activation and subsequent formation of IL-1β and IL-18. It exerts various other actions also like lowering of body temperature, increased sensitivity to central depressants, and depression of respiratory center. Colchicine is also used in management of chronic gout as bridging therapy with uric acid synthesis inhibitors to prevent development of symptoms of acute gouty arthritis initially due to mobilization of urate from tissues.

a. **Pharmacokinetics**: It has a rapid but variable absorption via oral route with no effect of food on its absorption. It achieves peak plasma concentrations within 0.5–2 hours. It is 39% plasma protein bound; larger volume of distribution due to formation of colchicine-tubulin complexes with different tissues and undergoes enterohepatic circulation accounting for its longer t1/2, i.e., 31 hours. It is metabolized mainly by oxidative demethylation with the help of enzyme CYP3A4. Approximately 40–65% of colchicine is excreted unchanged in urine, and the main organs with high colchicine concentration are the kidney, spleen, and liver sparing the heart, skeletal muscles, and brain. Colchicine acts as a substrate for P-glycoprotein efflux and is contraindicated in patients with hepatic or renal impairment already on CYP3A4 or P-glycoprotein inhibitor therapy.

b. **Dosage**: Individualization needs to be performed as per the age, renal/hepatic function, and concomitant medications and is administered only by oral route. A gap of 7–14 days should be present between courses of gout treatment with colchicine therapy to avoid accumulation of drug and further toxicity. Patients suffering from cardiac, hepatic, or renal disease are better off with NSAIDs or glucocorticoids. For the treatment of acute gout flare, two tablets 0.6 mg each should be taken first followed by a single 0.6 mg tablet after 1 hour. Pain, swelling, and redness subside within 12 hours and are resolved by 48–72 hours.

For prophylaxis in patients with recurrent gout having less than one attack per year, 0.6 mg tablet is to be taken 3 or 4 days per week; those having more than 1 attack per year, 0.6 mg tablet is to be taken daily; and those having severe attacks, 0.6 mg tablets are to be taken twice daily. Caution is to be taken in patients with hepatic or renal mutilation as the drug cannot be removed by hemodialysis.

c. **Adverse effects**: The most common adverse effects are gastrointestinal (nausea, vomiting, diarrhea, and abdominal pain) as the drug undergoes enterohepatic circulation and is in constant state of contact with gastric mucosa. It is advised to stop the drug on emergence of these symptoms. Other adverse effects include myelosuppression, leucopenia, granulocytopenia, neutropenia, aplastic anemia, and rhabdomyolysis [3–5, 11].

3. **Corticosteroids**: They provide symptomatic relief to a patient of acute gout during attacks and prevent further attacks by their anti-inflammatory action. They are mostly indicated in patients who cannot be prescribed NSAIDs and colchicine. Glucocorticoids provide their anti-inflammatory effect by various mechanisms: (a) induce production of lipocortin which inhibits phospholipase A2 and decreases production of arachidonic acid leading to decrease in synthesis of inflammatory mediators like prostaglandins, leukotrienes, and platelet-activating factor; (b) inhibit synthesis and release of cytokines (IL-1, IL-4, IL-6, and TNF-α) with reduced activation of T cells and fibroblast proliferation, thereby reducing process of chemotaxis; and (c) inhibit pro-inflammatory transcription factors like nuclear factor-κB and activating protein which leads to decreased enhancement of transcription of genes for COX-2, cytokines, and nitric oxide synthase (iNOS). The drugs used are prednisolone, methylprednisolone, and triamcinolone with the advantage of being given by oral route, intravenous route, or intra-articular administration.

a. Pharmacokinetics: All these three have an intermediate duration of action (12–36 hours). They are 90% plasma protein bound. They mainly bind to corticosteroid-binding globulin. They are metabolized both at hepatic and extrahepatic sites.

b. Dosage: Prednisolone is given in a dose of 40–60 mg per day orally or 40 mg per day intravenously. They are given at the initial dose for 2–5 days and then tapered over 7–10 days. Triamcinolone is given intra-articularly at a dose of 10–40 mg depending on the size of the joint. They should be taken early morning so as to have less effect of hypothalamic-pituitary axis suppression.

c. Adverse effects: They are an extension of their pharmacological actions seen with extended therapy. The adverse effects include altered distribution of fat throughout the body, edema, hypokalemia, hypertension, suppression of hypothalamic-pituitary axis, osteoporosis, hyperglycemia, peptic ulcer, cataract formation, glaucoma, myopathy, muscle wasting, susceptibility to infections, and central nervous system (CNS) side effects like psychiatric disturbances, acne, weight gain, and hyperlipidemia [4, 12].

5.2.2 For chronic gout

1. **Uricosurics**: These are drugs which favor excretion of uric acid from the body.

a. **Probenecid**: It is a highly lipid-soluble benzoic acid derivative. It mainly acts by inhibiting transport of organic acids across the epithelial barrier. Reabsorption of uric acid is inhibited by its action on the organic anion transporters (OAT) mainly urate transporter-1 (URAT-1). In addition, it also hampers pharmacokinetic properties of many other drugs also, i.e., retards tubular secretion of methotrexate and active metabolite of clofibrate, inhibits renal secretion of inactive glucuronide metabolites of naproxen, ketoprofen, and indomethacin thereby increasing their plasma concentration, hampers transport of drugs such as penicillin G, and raises the plasma levels of β lactam.

   i. Pharmacokinetics: Complete absorption occurs after oral administration and attains peak plasma concentrations within 2–4 hours. It has a dose-dependent $t_{1/2}$ and varies between less than 5 to more than 8 hours. It is 85–95% bound to plasma albumin, and the unbound part is excreted by glomerular filtration and active tubular secretion.

   ii. Dosage: Initially it is given in a dose of 250 mg twice daily and increased over 1–2 weeks to 500–1000 mg twice daily. Patient should be advised to increase the daily water intake to prevent formation of renal stones as probenecid increases urinary urate levels. De-escalation is to be started after 6 months of treatment if the uric acid levels are favorable.

   iii. Adverse effects: Mild gastrointestinal irritation is mostly seen and that too with higher doses. It should be avoided in patients with creatinine clearance 50 ml/min and is also ineffective in these patients. Overdosage leads to CNS stimulation, convulsions, and death due to respiratory failure. It is contraindicated in patients with history of renal stones [13, 14].

b. **Sulfinpyrazone**: It has neither analgesic nor neither anti-inflammatory property. It inhibits tubular reabsorption of uric acid. Due to its higher incidence of gastric irritation and other side effects, it is not used nowadays [15].

c. **Benzbromarone**: It is a reversible urate anion exchanger inhibitor present in the proximal tubule. It has not been approved by the United States (US) Food and Drug Administration (FDA) due to its risk of causing severe hepatotoxicity; however, it is used as a potent uricosuric in certain Southeast Asian countries [16].

d. **Lesinurad**: Another uricosuric which has been approved for use in combination therapy with a xanthine oxidase inhibitor. It acts by inhibiting the transporters URAT-1 and OAT-4 and decreasing reabsorption of uric acid.

   i. Pharmacokinetics: It has a fast oral absorption showing 100% availability and is largely plasma protein bound. It has a t1/2 of 5 hours, metabolized by CYP2C9, and is excreted in urine and feces.

   ii. Dosage: Given at a dosage of 200 mg per day along with a xanthine oxidase inhibitor. It should not be used in patients with creatinine clearance 45 ml/min.

iii. Adverse effects: Black box warning has been issued by the US FDA against its use as monotherapy due to risk of causing acute renal failure. It has also propensity to cause an increase in serum creatinine levels. Other adverse effects like headache and gastritis can also occur. Interruption with xanthine oxidase inhibitor requires stoppage of lesinurad also [14].

2. **Uric acid synthesis inhibitors (Xanthine oxidase inhibitors)**

a. **Allopurinol**: This compound was initially produced as an antineoplastic agent and was later found to lack that property. Later it was found to have xanthine oxidase enzyme-inhibiting property. Xanthine oxidase enzyme is responsible for conversion of hypoxanthine and xanthine into urate, and by inhibiting this enzyme, allopurinol prevents formation of urate. Allopurinol in low concentrations acts as a competitive and as a noncompetitive inhibitor at high concentrations of xanthine oxidase enzyme. The formation of oxypurinol (alloxanthine), its primary metabolite, and its long perseverance in tissues is majorly responsible for its activity. Oxypurinol inhibits the reduced form of xanthine oxidase enzyme. Conversion of hypoxanthine to xanthine takes place in the presence of xanthine oxidase enzyme which is also blocked by allopurinol (inhibition of de novo purine synthesis). The purines are mainly excreted by the kidney. In the absence of allopurinol, the major purine excreted is uric acid, whereas it is hypoxanthine, xanthine, and uric acid in the presence of allopurinol. This treatment leads to excess purine load in the kidney which might lead to a risk of xanthine stones which can be minimized by increasing the fluid intake and alkalization of urine. It also helps in dissolution of tophi and decreases the chances of development and progression of chronic gouty arthritis. It also prevents development of nephropathy by preventing formation of uric acid stones; however, it cannot restore the renal function after injury to the renal tissue has occurred, but it may retard the progression. Initially on starting the therapy, chances of acute attack of gouty arthritis increase due to movement of uric acid outside from the tissues, and this can be concealed by giving NSAIDs and colchicine along with allopurinol. Allopurinol is also used in patients undergoing chemotherapy for hematological malignancies to prevent hyperuricemia and consequently gout.

i. Pharmacokinetics: It has a fast oral absorption with peak plasma concentrations achieved in 60–90 min. Plasma half-life of allopurinol is 1–2 hours and that of oxypurinol is 18–30 hours which allows for once daily dosing. It undergoes metabolism which leads to formation of its metabolite oxypurinol. Around 20% of unabsorbed drug is excreted in feces within 48–72 hours, and other 10–30% of unabsorbed drug is excreted in urine. It is not bound to any plasma protein and is distributed in total tissue water except the brain. Oxypurinol is excreted via glomerular filtration.

ii. Dosage: It can be given both as an oral and intravenous preparation. The main aim of treatment is to decrease the uric acid level to 6 mg/dl. The drug is initially started at 100 mg/day for patients with glomerular filtration >40 mg/min and is increased by 100 mg weekly. It is usually given in once daily dosing, but dosing above 300 mg should be divided accordingly. Dosage in patients with reduced glomerular filtration (<40 mg/min) should be less than that of a normal person (>60 mg/min).

iii. Adverse effects: It is generally well tolerated. However, the most common adverse effects are hypersensitivity reactions which are seen after months and years of treatment, and this can further precipitate into serious reactions if the drug is not stopped. The cutaneous reactions seen are mainly pruritic, erythematous, or maculopapular eruption. It is contraindicated in patients who previously have experienced serious reactions with it, in nursing mothers and in children except those with malignancy and inborn errors of metabolism. It increases half-life of probenecid and enhances its uricosuric effect; on the other hand, probenecid increases clearance of oxypurinol, thereby increasing the dose required. Allopurinol also inhibits enzymatic activation of mercaptopurine and azathioprine by xanthine oxidase enzyme which should be kept in mind in patients undergoing chemotherapy. It also increases risk of bone marrow suppression if given with cytotoxic drugs and interferes with metabolic inactivation of some drugs like warfarin.

b. **Febuxostat**: Another xanthine oxidase inhibitor which has been approved for treatment of hyperuricemia in gout though it is not recommended for treatment of asymptomatic hyperuricemia, having the advantage of being more potent, selective, no dose reduction in renal disease patients, and less chances of causing allergic reactions. Febuxostat is used in conditions when patient is intolerant to allopurinol or when it is contraindicated. It is a non-purine inhibitor of xanthine oxidase enzyme inhibiting both reduced and oxidized forms of the enzyme. It usually requires concurrent treatment with NSAIDs or colchicine.

i. Pharmacokinetics: It has a rapid absorption with peak plasma concentrations being achieved after 1–1.5 hours of drug intake. The half-life is around 5–8 hours and is metabolized both by conjugation by UGT enzymes (UGT1A1, UGT1A3, UGT1A9, and UGT2B7) and oxidized by CYP enzymes (CYP1A2, CYP2C8, CYP2C9) and non-CYP enzymes indicating possibility of drug-drug interactions. It is excreted by both hepatic and renal routes. No dose reduction is required in case of mild to moderate hepatic or renal impairment.

ii. Dosage: It is initiated at 40 mg/day and is increased as per the patient's uric acid levels.

iii. Adverse effects: The most common adverse effect seen with it is abnormality with liver function tests, nausea, joint pain, and rash, so regular monitoring of liver function is required. It can also cause an increase in gout flares as during the therapy there is mobilization of urate crystals from the tissue deposits due to a decrease in the uric acid levels. Patients should also be regularly checked for any cardiovascular complications. Drug levels of theophylline, mercaptopurine, and azathioprine, which are metabolized by xanthine oxidase enzyme, are increased if given with febuxostat and febuxostat and are contraindicated in patients taking azathioprine or mercaptopurine.

3. **Uricase**: It is an enzyme which is present in birds which converts uric acid into soluble allantoin which is easily excreted.

a. **Rasburicase**: A recombinant uricase which has been shown to lower urate levels much efficiently than allopurinol. It has been indicated as the initial management for elevated uric acid levels in children and adults suffering from leukemia, lymphoma, and solid tumor malignancies and undergoing chemotherapy leading to significant hyperuricemia. However, there are certain limitations with it like formations of antibodies against it.

   i. Dosage: It is given as 0.2 mg/kg IV as infusion over 30 minutes every day up to 5 days.

   ii. Adverse effects: Certain adverse effects like nausea, headache, constipation, diarrhea, hemolysis in glucose-6-phosphate dehydrogenase (G6PD) deficient patients, methemoglobinemia, acute renal failure, and anaphylaxis are seen with it.

b. **Pegloticase**: It is pegylated uricase converting uric acid into soluble allantoin. It is used for the treatment of severe, treatment refractory, chronic gout or when other urate-lowering therapies are contraindicated. Problem of development of antibodies against it is seen with pegloticase also.

   i. Dosage: It is administered at 8 mg every 2 weeks as an infusion.

   ii. Adverse effects: Vomiting, nausea, chest pain, constipation, diarrhea, erythema, pruritis, urticaria, hemolysis in G6PD deficient patients, and anaphylaxis are certain adverse effects seen with it. Black box warning has been issued by US FDA against pegloticase which advises that the drug should only be administered in health-care settings and only by health-care professionals to manage anaphylactic reactions and other serious reactions [11, 17].

6. Recent developments

a. **Arhalofenate:** It has been synthesized showing a dual mechanism of action but is still pending in approval. It acts as a partial agonist to peroxisome proliferator-activated receptor-γ (PPAR-γ) and inhibits expression of IL-1, thereby inhibiting renal absorption of uric acid in the kidney by URAT-1, OAT-4, and OAT-10 transporters [18].It was initially synthesized as a drug for the management of type 2 diabetes mellitus but was also found to have anti-flare and uricosuric property. Its phase II study has been completed showing positive results, and further results from ongoing studies are awaited [19].

b. **Interleukin-1 inhibitors (anakinra, canakinumab, rilonacept):** These prevent attraction of neutrophils at the joint site. The drugs in this class are anakinra, an interleukin-1 receptor antagonist; canakinumab, a monoclonal antibody against interleukin-1 beta; and rilonacept, a chimera constituting of IgG domains and extracellular components of interleukin-1 receptor. All these have been shown to have efficacy in acute gout but still have not been approved by the drug regulatory authorities [7]. However, these are approved for their use in other diseases like rheumatoid arthritis and cryptoporphyrin-associated periodic syndrome. They are contraindicated in patients with previous hypersensitivity reactions to these drugs and any serious active infection. Further application concomitant live attenuated vaccine is to be avoided. Concern of immunosuppression with their use has been an important reason for their disapproval [20].

c. **Verinurad:** It is also a uricosuric which inhibits the reabsorption of uric acid by acting on the URAT-1. It has been shown to be 3 times more potent than benzbromarone and 100 times more potent than probenecid and has completed phase II clinical trial.

d. **Tranilast:** It is a moderately sedative H1 anihistaminic drug, which is used in management of bronchial asthma and other allergic conditions in Japan. It has also been shown to reduce serum uric acid levels by inhibition of URAT-1 transporter and promoting excretion of urate. In addition, it has also been shown to decrease the inflammation induced by monosodium crystals in vivo by reducing leukocyte infiltration and plasma extravasation similar to colchicine and indomethacin, thereby causing flare reduction. It has completed its phase II clinical trial.

e. **Levotofisopam:** It is an S-enantiomer of racemic tofisopam which is a benzodiazepine derivative which has been approved in the United States for the management of anxiety. Phase I clinical trial has been completed, phase II studies are underway, and results are awaited.

f. **Topiroxostat:** It is a selective xanthine oxidase inhibitor. Its mechanism of action is different from that of febuxostat such that it acts as a hybrid inhibitor. It not only acts as a chemical structure based xanthine oxidase enzyme inhibition but also covalently binds to molybdenum in the active center during the hydroxylation process of the enzyme. The pharmacokinetics of topiroxostat is unaltered by mild to moderate renal impairment. It has a half-life of around 20 hours, and enzyme activity takes time to recover even after the drug has been metabolized. In patients with concurrent moderate renal impairment and hyperuricemia, a fall in serum urate and albumin levels has been reported. It has been approved by the Pharmaceuticals and Medical Devices Agency, in Japan in the year 2013, in a dose of 20–80 mg twice daily.

g. **Ulodesine:** It acts by inhibiting purine nucleotide phosphorylase (PNP) which is an enzyme that acts one-step before xanthine oxidase in production of urate. Initial concerns were shown due to inhibition of PNP enzyme due to its absence in immunodeficient patients and in patients suffering from immunologic disorders, but nothing has been reported in studies until date. Phase II studies have been completed, and further studies are awaited [19].

We all authors share the opinion that therapy of the chronic tophaceous gout is still far from optimal. Despite availability of several agents, none has been considered as ideal due either to their undesirable adverse effects profile, limited utility in patients of renal impairment, inadequate response or failure to reverse existing osseous lesions, and dissolution of tophi from the tissues. We anticipate that newer drugs that are being developed with different mechanism of actions might address these issues, but only time will prove their worth.

7. Conclusions

Gout is a metabolic disorder due to the rise in uric acid levels in the body leading to development of gouty arthritis. Its management requires both pharmacological and non-pharmacological intervention. Newer drugs targeting various inflammatory mediators, enzymes, or transporters are in different phases of clinical development. Until date, none has reached to phase III and yet to get an approval from regulatory bodies. The quest for an optimally designed drug with desirable efficacy and acceptable safety profile is still on.

Acknowledgements

We would like to thank Dr. Rajesh Kumar, Dr. Ketan Patil, and Dr. Preetish Kumar Panigrahy (Senior Residents, Department of Pharmacology, AIIMS, Jodhpur, India) and Dr. Govind Mishra, Dr. Ravi Prakash Sharma, and Dr. Sameer Khasbage (Junior Residents, Department of Pharmacology, AIIMS, Jodhpur, India) for their help and support, whenever needed.

Conflict of interest

None.

Funding

This chapter is non-funded.

Acronyms and abbreviations

CNS	central nervous system
COX	cyclooxygenase
G6PD	glucose-6-phosphate dehydrogenase
IL	interleukin
iNOS	nitric oxide synthase
NSAIDs	nonsteroidal anti-inflammatory drugs
OAT	organic anion transporters
PNP	purine nucleotide phosphorylase
t1/2	half-life
TNF	tumor necrosis factor
URAT	urate transporter

Author details

Rajit Sahai, Pramod Kumar Sharma*, Arup Misra and Siddhartha Dutta
Department of Pharmacology, All India Institute of Medical Sciences,
Jodhpur, India

*Address all correspondence to: pramod309@gmail.com

References

[1] Schumacher HR, Chen LX. Gout and other crystal associated arthropathies. In: Kasper DL, Fauci AS, Hauser SL, Longo DL, Jameson JL, Loscalzo J, editors. Harrison's principles of internal medicine. 19th ed. United States of America: Mc Graw Hill Education; 2015. p. 2233

[2] Kuo CF, Grainge MJ, Zhang W, Doherty M. Global epidemiology of gout: Prevalence, incidence and risk factors. Nature Reviews Rheumatology. 2015;**11**:649-662

[3] Grosser T, Smyth EM, FitzGerald GA. Pharmacotherapy of inflammation, pain, fever and gout. In: Dandan RH, Knollmann BC. 13th ed. Goodman and Gillman's the pharmacological basis of therapeutics. United States of America: Mc Graw Hill Education; 2018:702

[4] Hellmann DB, Imboden JB. Rheumatologic, immunologic and allergic disorders. In: Papadakis MA, SJ MP, editors. Current medical diagnosis and treatment. 58th ed. United States of America: Mc Graw Hill Education; 2019. p. 844

[5] Hellmann DB, Imboden JB. Rheumatologic, immunologic and allergic disorders. In: Papadakis MA, SJ MP, editors. Current medical diagnosis and treatment. 58th ed. United States of America: Mc Graw Hill Education; 2019. p. 845

[6] Schumacher HR, Chen LX. Gout and other crystal associated arthropathies. In: Kasper DL, Fauci AS, Hauser SL, Longo DL, Jameson JL, Loscalzo J. 19th ed. Harrison's principles of internal medicine. United States of America: Mc Graw Hill Education; 2015:2234

[7] Hellmann DB, Imboden JB. Rheumatologic, immunologic and allergic disorders. In: Papadakis MA, SJ MP, editors. Current medical diagnosis and treatment. 58th ed. United States of America: Mc Graw Hill Education; 2019. p. 846

[8] Grosser T, Smyth EM, FitzGerald GA. Pharmacotherapy of inflammation, pain, fever and gout. In: Dandan RH, Knollmann BC. 13th ed. Goodman and Gillman's the pharmacological basis of therapeutics. United States of America: Mc Graw Hill Education; 2018:698-699

[9] Grosser T, Smyth EM, GA FG. Pharmacotherapy of inflammation, pain, fever and gout. In: Dandan RH, Knollmann BC, editors. Goodman and Gillman's the pharmacological basis of therapeutics. 13th ed. United States of America: Mc Graw Hill Education; 2018. pp. 700-701

[10] Grosser T, Smyth EM, GA FG. Pharmacotherapy of inflammation, pain, fever and gout. In: Dandan RH, Knollmann BC, editors. Goodman and Gillman's the pharmacological basis of therapeutics. 13th ed. United States of America: Mc Graw Hill Education; 2018. p. 697

[11] Grosser T, Smyth EM, GA FG. Pharmacotherapy of inflammation, pain, fever and gout. In: Dandan RH, Knollmann BC, editors. Goodman and Gillman's the pharmacological basis of therapeutics. 13th ed. United States of America: Mc Graw Hill Education; 2018. p. 703

[12] Grosser T, Smyth EM, FitzGerald GA. Adrenocorticotropic hormone, adrenal steroids, and the adrenal cortex. In: Dandan RH, Knollmann BC. 13th ed. Goodman and Gillman's the pharmacological basis of therapeutics. United States of America: Mc Graw Hill Education; 2018:852-855

[13] Hellmann DB, Imboden JB. Rheumatologic, immunologic and allergic disorders. In: Papadakis MA, SJ

MP, editors. Current medical diagnosis and treatment. 58th ed. United States of America: Mc Graw Hill Education; 2019. p. 847

[14] Grosser T, Smyth EM, GA FG. Pharmacotherapy of inflammation, pain, fever and gout. In: Dandan RH, Knollmann BC, editors. Goodman and Gillman's the pharmacological basis of therapeutics. 13th ed. United States of America: Mc Graw Hill Education; 2018. pp. 705-706

[15] Tripathi KD. Antirheumatoid and antigout drugs. In: Tripathi M, editor. Essential's of Medical Pharmacology. 8th ed. India: Jaypeebrothers medical publishers ltd; 2018. p. 233

[16] Terkeltaub R. Emerging uricosurics for gout. Expert Review of Clinical Pharmacology. 2017;**10**(3):247-249

[17] Grosser T, Smyth EM, GA FG. Pharmacotherapy of inflammation, pain, fever and gout. In: Dandan RH, Knollmann BC, editors. Goodman and Gillman's the pharmacological basis of therapeutics. 13th ed. United States of America: Mc Graw Hill Education; 2018. pp. 704-705

[18] Igel TF, Krasnokutsky S, Pillinger MH. Recent advances in understanding and managing gout. F1000 Research. 2017;**6**(F1000 faculty rev):1-11

[19] Satuii SE, Gaffo AL. Treatment of hyperuricemia in gout: Current therapeutic options, latest developments and clinical implications. Therapeutic Advances in Musculoskeletal Disease. 2016;**8**(4):145-159

[20] Grosser T, Smyth EM, GA FG. Pharmacotherapy of inflammation, pain, fever and gout. In: Dandan RH, Knollmann BC, editors. Goodman and Gillman's the pharmacological basis of therapeutics. 13th ed. United States of America: Mc Graw Hill Education; 2018. p. 648

Chapter 4

Personalized Medicine of Urate-Lowering Therapy for Gout

Dewen Yan and Youming Zhang

Abstract

Gout is a common and complex form of arthritis that is characterized with hyperuricaemia. It is required urate-lowering therapy (ULT) for lifelong management. ULT includes decreasing uric acid product in serum, increasing renal urate excretion and promoting uric acid to allantoin for excretion. Whole genome association studies in gout identified more than 40 genetic loci that influenced the serum uric acid levels. Most associated genes were found to affect renal urate excretion. Pharmacogenetics and pharmacogenomics approaches on ULT had revealed several genes that underlined the effectiveness and the adverse events of medications for gout. Together with the researches on epigenetic factors such as DNA methylations, miRNAs; and the discovery of environmental factors such as microbiota and metabolites, the current progress provides the opportunities for personalized management of ULT for treating hyperuricaemia and gout.

Keywords: gout, hyperuricaemia, pharmacogenetics, pharmacogenomics, urate-lowering therapy

1. Introduction

The term "gout" was firstly used around 1200 AD. It means "a drop" of liquid from the Latin word gutta [1]. The first description of gout as a disease was from Egypt in 2600 BC as arthritis of the big toe. Gout is now referred as a form of inflammatory arthritis characterized by recurrent attacks of a red, tender, hot, and swollen joint [2]. It is one of the most common forms of arthritis and the prevalence is increasing worldwide. The prevalence is various in different regions across the world and is about 1–4%. In westernized countries, the prevalence is about 3–6% in men and about 1–2% in women. Prevalence can increase up to 10% in some countries. For people aged more than 80 years old, it could rise up to 10% in men and 6% in women [3, 4]. In the USA, the prevalence of gout in adults was estimated to be approximately 3.9% [5]. From 1990 to 2015, the number of prevalent gout cases rose by 30% in Nordic region [6]. In China, the pooled prevalence of gout was 1.1% between 2000 and 2016 [7].

Hyperuricaemia is the key biochemical abnormality in gout. Uric acid is a $C_5H_4N_4O_3$ (7,9-dihydro-1H-purine-2,6,8(3H)-trione) heterocyclic organic compound with a molecular weight of 168 Da. Uric acid is the product from the conversion of the two purine nucleic acids, adenine and guanine [8]. Hyperuricaemia is defined as serum urate level more than 0.42 mmol/l. It results in the formation of monosodium urate (MSU) crystals. MSU crystals precipitate within joints and soft tissues to cause an inflammatory response. The prominent clinical features of gout are attacks of tendonitis, formatting collections of MSU crystals as tophi, joint destruction and chronic gouty arthritis. MSU crystals can also deposit in the interstitium of the kidneys to form renal stones. Hyperuricaemia was associated with hypertension and ischemic heart diseases [9, 10]. The causes of hyperuricaemia are either under excretion of uric acid in the kidneys or increase of production of uric acid in serum [11]. Two key enzymes regulate the production of uric acid. One is xanthine oxidase that makes xanthine to uric acid; the other is urate oxidase that transfers uric acid to allantoin. Allantoin is the end product of purine catabolism in all mammals except humans, great apes, and one breed of dog, the Dalmatian. An animal model of hyperuricaemia from Dalmatian dog revealed the importance of *SLC2A9* gene for uric acid transport in mammals [12]. Together with renal excretion of uric acid, these are three clinical management paths of uric acid to maintain the lower level of uric acid in serum. These include to decrease uric acid production (xanthine oxidase inhibitors—allopurinol, febuxostat), increase renal urate excretion (uricosurics—benzbromarone, probenecid, lesinurad), or promote uric acid to allantoin which is more water soluble and readily excreted (recombinant uricases—pegloticase) [11]. Environmental factors and genetic factors are the major causes to influence the drugs' efficiencies and side effects for gout.

2. Clinical managements of gout

Effective treatment of acute gout attacks and long-term urate lowering therapy are clinical managements of gout. An acute attack should be treated as soon as possible with non-steroidal anti-inflammatory drugs (NSAIDs) or colchicine as first line treatment options. For patients who do not respond NSAIDs or colchicine, systemic corticosteroids generally are applied [13]. Long-term management of gout with ULT is required for patients who are confirmed as diagnosis of gout and tophi. The diagnosis includes more than two times gout attacks per year, renal stones or stage 2 or worse chronic kidney disease. A sustained reduction of serum urate to less than 0.36 mmol/l (6 mg/dl) is generally recommended and a lower target of less than 0.30 mmol/l (5 mg/dl) is recommended in patients with tophi [14, 15]. A xanthine oxidase inhibitor is the recommended as first-line choice for ULT. A uricosuric can be serviced as second-line medication for ULT. It is for patients who do not response xanthine oxidase inhibitors well. Uricases are the third-line treatments for patients who have refractory disease and are intolerant to oral ULTs. Optimizing therapy for improving the outcomes with affordable drugs such as allopurinol, as well as rationalizing the use of new, more expensive agents is an important clinical goal. The roles of pharmacogenetics and pharmacogenomics are becoming more and more important to predict drug response and adverse events of medications. Rationalization and combination of common medications with genetic screening and other environmental factors will revolutionize gout managements in near future.

3. Pharmacogenetics and pharmacogenomics in ULT

"Pharmacogenetics" was a term originally to describe clinical observations of inherited differences in drug effects in 1950s [16]. It is now defined as the study of individual DNA variants that are related to drug responses [17, 18]. Genetic variants also underlie the differential susceptibility to diseases and the sensitivity to drug adverse events. Most drug effects are determined by the interplay of several proteins that influence the pharmacokinetics and pharmacodynamics of medications, including inherited differences in drug targets such as receptors, drug disposition such as metabolizing enzymes and transporters, drug metabolism, and drug adverse reaction. In human, about 20–95% of variability in drug disposition and effects are determined by genetic polymorphisms in the genome [18]. For all practical purpose, the terms pharmacogenetics and pharmacogenomics may be synonymous, but pharmacogenomics normally refers genome-wide approaches to investigate all genes in the genome that influence drug responses while pharmacogenetics implies the study of a single gene's interactions with drugs. The pharmacogenomics approach tends to be applied to identify genes in the search for novel drug targets. This is in contrast to traditional drug design that depends on a prior knowledge of the target and is based on high-throughput screening to identify small-molecule antagonists or agonists.

3.1 Genetic and genomic approaches of hyperuricaemia and gout

Genetic approaches for complicated diseases and associated traits such as gout and hyperuricaemia are to identify genetic variants in genome that underlie the diseases and syndromes. There are many kinds of genetic variants in human genome. Single nuclear polymorphisms (SNPs) are the most frequent variants found in the genome, accounting for 90% of human genetic variation. Total 84.7 million SNPs were found in 26 human populations [19]. SNPs can be found within coding sequences and noncoding regions of genes, as well as within intergenic regions. Insertion and deletion of short segments of DNA (INDEL) is another type of common polymorphism. More than 3.6 million short insertions/deletions are distributed throughout the human genome, with approximately 36% of them being located within promoters, introns, and exons of known genes [19, 20]. They can have a significant impact on gene function not only when present in exonic coding sequence but also when within a gene intron [21]. Variable number of tandem repeats (VNTRs) polymorphisms is widespread in the genome and contain variable numbers of repeated nucleotide sequences that result in alleles of varying lengths. VNTR loci typically have high levels of heterozygosity that make them very informative for genetics research. There are about 60,000 structural variants around human genome [19]. Inversions may involve larger regions of the genome in which a segment of a chromosome is reversed end to end and occur when a chromosome breaks in two places. A copy number variant (CNV) is a segment of DNA for which there are more than two copies in the genome. The genetic segment involved may range from one kilobase to several megabases in size [22]. Many techniques can allow the detection and discovery of CNVs including cytogenetic techniques such as fluorescent in situ hybridization, comparative genomic hybridization, array comparative genomic hybridization, and by large-scale SNP genotyping.

The genetic approaches to hyperuricaemia and gout include candidate gene studies, positional cloning studies and genome-wide association studies (GWASs). Candidate gene study needs to have relatively big case and control groups to increase the power for statistical analysis. Positional cloning is another genetic approach that identifies disease genes by progressive dissection of linkage regions that are consistently co-inherited with the disease. Nowadays, GWASs have been rapidly changing the landscape of the search of the genes that underlie complicated diseases such as hyperuricaemia and gout. It is a powerful approach to overcome the limitations of candidate gene and positional cloning studies. It examines the relationships between allele frequencies and disease status or associated traits with a large number of genetic polymorphism markers covering of whole genome [23]. GWASs provide the opportunity to identify novel mechanisms of disease pathogenesis that are caused by previously unsuspected genes or regulatory regions. About 10,000 strong associations have been reported between genetic variants and one or more complex traits [24].

3.2 GWASs for hyperuricaemia and gout

More than 30 GWASs papers on hyperuricaemia and gout have been published so far. The first GWAS study identified the associations of three genetic loci with uric acid concentration and risk of gout [25]. The three loci were *SLC2A9*, *ABCG2* and *SLC17A3*. Since then, many GWSs papers have been published across the world and discovered more than 40 genes that showed the associations with hyperuricaemia or gout. Many genes identified by GWASs encode urate transporters and interacting proteins. The identified genetic variation can only explain less than 10% level of variance for serum uric acid levels [26]. The rest could be explained by environmental factors and the interactions of genetic factors and environmental factors. We listed 10 genes that were frequently identified in GWASs studies worldwide in **Table 1** and also discussed the genes' potential function roles in regulating uric acid metabolism in serum.

3.2.1 SLC2A9

SLC2A9 was a gene that was identified in almost every GWAS across the world. The gene is located on human chromosome 4p16 and encodes a member of the

Genes	Encoded protein	Chr.	Ref.	Populations	Possible function roles
SLC2A9	Solute carrier family 2 member 9: GLUT9	4p16	[25, 27–37]	African, Asian, European	Regulating renal and gut excretion of uric acid
ABCG2	ATP binding cassette subfamily G member 2	4q22	[25, 29, 30, 33, 35, 36, 45]	Asian, European	Regulating extra-renal uric acid under-excretion
SLC17A cluster	Sodium phosphate transporters	6p22	[25, 33, 35, 45]	Asian, European	Regulating renal and excretion of uric acid
GCKR	SIS (Sugar ISomerase) family protein	2p23	[33, 35, 45]	Asian, European	Regulating glucokinase in cells
SLC22A cluster	Integral membrane proteins	11q12	[28–30, 33, 35, 45]	African, Asian, European	Preventing potentially harmful organic anions
PDZK1	PDZ domain-containing scaffolding protein	1q21	[33, 35, 36]	Asian, European	Regulating the high-density lipoproteins
INHBC and INHBE	TGF-beta superfamily of proteins	12q13	[33, 45]	Asian, European	Regulating numerous cellular processes
A1CF	APOBEC1 complementation factor	10q11	[33, 35]	Asian, European	Regulating RNA-binding subunit
MAF	Leucine zipper-containing transcription factor	16q23	[30, 33]	Asian, European	Regulating several cellular processes
SLC16A9	Solute carrier family 16 member 9	10q21	[33, 35]	Asian, European	Regulating monocarboxylic acid transporter

Chr: chromosome; Ref: reference.

Table 1.
The 10 most replicated genes in GWAS studies for hyperruricemia and gout.

SLC2A facilitative glucose transporter family GLUT-9. The associations with hyperuricaemia and gout were found in populations from Africa American, Asia, Europe and the United States [25, 27–37], but not found in Hispanic American [38]. Variation in *SLC2A9* was the most statistically significant genetic determinant of serum urate; accounting for 3.4–8.8% of the variance in women and 0.5–2.0% of the variance in men [25, 31, 34, 37, 39, 40]. The encoded protein is involved in p21-activated protein kinase (PAK) pathway for transport of glucose, bile salts, organic acids, metal ions and amine compounds. Recent studies showed that GLUT-9 was participated in renal and gut excretion of uric acid and was implicated in antioxidant defense [41–43]. There are two distinct N-terminal isoforms of human GLUT-9: GLUT-9a (540 residues) and GLUT-9b (511 residues) [44]. These isoforms are generated by alternative splicing of 5′ ends and differ in membrane trafficking. GLUT-9b has a more substantial role in urate homeostasis than GLUT-9a. GLUT-9a is likely to function as the exit site for urate from proximal tubule cells, whereas GLUT-9b might transport urate into the proximal tubule cells across the apical membrane [26].

3.2.2 ABCG2

ABCG2 gene is located in human chromosome 4q22. It encodes ATP binding cassette subfamily G member 2. ABC proteins transport various molecules across extra- and intra-cellular membranes. The gene was also found to have associations with hyperuricaemia and gout in Asian, European and the United States [25, 29, 30, 33, 35, 36, 45]. The gene product is involved primarily in extra-renal uric acid under-excretion. Multiple transcript variants encoding different isoforms had been found for this gene [46]. ABCG2 is expressed in the brush border membrane of the proximal tubules of the kidney and has a role in the apical [47]. The ABCG2 Q141 K variant is highly likely to be causal and results in internalization of *ABCG2*, which can be rescued by drugs [48]. The SNP rs2231142 in *ABCG2* gene had significant associations between gout and controls, between gout and hyperuricaemia, and between hyperuricaemia and controls, respectively. In a cell model investigation it showed significantly higher IL-8 release from endothelial cell (EC) combined with *ABCG2* knockdown [49]. The Glu141Lys polymorphism was accounted for 0.57% of the variation in serum urate from a meta-analysis of GWAS data [35]. The polymorphism had a significantly larger effect on serum urate levels in men than in women. The Glu141Lys substitution was shown that it caused a 53% reduction in the rate of ABCG2-assocaited urate transport [35]. The polymorphism of the gene could also affect the response to allopurinol [50].

3.2.3 SCL17A gene cluster

SCL17A gene cluster is located on human chromosome 6p21 containing three members of the *SLC17* gene family (*SLC17A3, SLC17A1* and *SLC17A4*). The polymorphisms of the genes were identified as a significant predictor of uric acid levels and gout in many GWASs [25, 33, 35, 45]. The strongest association was with SNP rs1165205 within intron 1 of *SLC17A3*. The *SLC17A3* gene encodes a sodium phosphate transporter (NPT4) which is expressed at the apical membrane of renal proximal tubule cells. The *SLC17A1* gene lies immediately downstream of *SLC17A3* and encodes sodium phosphate transporter NPT1, which is expressed in the human kidney and can transport uric acid in vitro [51]. SNP rs1183201 within *SLC17A1* was identified as the strongest predictor of serum urate in a meta-analysis of GWAS [35]. Further investigations will be required to identify the causal SNPs in the gene cluster that regulate uric acid levels and susceptibility to gout [52].

3.2.4 GCKR

GCKR gene is located on human chromosome 2p23. The gene encodes a protein belonging to the glucokinase regulator (GCKR) subfamily. It inhibits glucokinase in liver and pancreatic islet cells by binding non-covalently to form an inactive complex. This gene is also considered a susceptibility candidate gene for a form of maturity-onset diabetes of the young (MODY) and it has been found to have association with gout or hyperuricaemia in many populations [25, 33, 35, 45].

3.2.5 SLC22A cluster

SLC22A cluster is located on human chromosome 11q13. The cluster contains *SLC22A11* and *SLC22A12*. The encoded proteins are involved in the sodium-independent transport and excretion of organic anions. They are integral membrane proteins and are found mainly in the kidney and in the placenta, where they may act to prevent potentially harmful organic anions from reaching the foetus. The cluster was found to have associations to hyperuricaemia and gout in many populations [28–30, 33, 35, 45]. Selected rare variants in SLC22A12 were validated in transport studies, confirming three as loss-of-function (R325W, R405C, and T467M) and providing the therapeutic potential of the new URAT1-blocker lesinurad [53].

3.2.6 PDZK1

PDZK1 gene is located on human chromosome 1q21. This gene encodes a protein containing a PDZ domain. It mediates the subcellular localization of target proteins. *PDZK1* mediates the localization of cell surface proteins and plays an important role in cholesterol metabolism by regulating the high-density lipoproteins (HDL) receptor. Alternatively spliced transcript variants encoding multiple isoforms have been observed for this gene. The gene was showed to have associations with gout and hyperuricaemia in many populations [33, 35, 36]. The maximally associated genetic variant SNP rs1967017 at the *PDZK1* locus was found to elevated *PDZK1* expression. Transcriptional factor hepatocyte nuclear factor 4 alpha (HNF4A) physically binds the rs1967017 region. The urate-raising T allele of rs1967017 enhances HNF4A binding to the *PDZK1* promoter to increase *PDZK1* expression [54].

3.2.7 INHBC and INHBE

The INHBC and INHBE genes are located on human chromosome 12q13. The genes encode members of the TGF-beta (transforming growth factor-beta) superfamily of proteins. These proteins were implicated in regulating numerous cellular processes including cell proliferation, apoptosis, immune response and hormone secretion. They may be upregulated under conditions of endoplasmic reticulum stress, and may inhibit cellular proliferation and growth in pancreas and liver. The GWAS investigation found the genes had associations with gout and hyperuricaemia in some populations [33, 45].

3.2.8 A1CF

The *A1CF* gene is located on human chromosome 10q11. The encoded protein has three non-identical RNA recognition motifs and belongs to the heterogeneous ribonucleoproteins (hnRNP) family of RNA-binding proteins. It has been proposed that this complementation factor functions as an RNA-binding subunit and docks APOBEC-1 to deaminate the upstream cytidine. Studies suggest that the protein may also be involved in other RNA editing or RNA processing events. Several transcript variants encoding a few different isoforms have been found for. This gene was showed to have associations with gout and hyperuricaemia in some populations [33, 35].

3.2.9 MAF

The *MAF* gene is located on human chromosome 16q23. The encoded protein is a DNA-binding, leucine zipper-containing transcription factor and acts as a homodimer or as a heterodimer. It plays a role in the regulation of cellular processes, development, apoptosis and chondrocyte differentiation. Two transcript variants encoding different isoforms have been found for this gene. The polymorphisms of the gene were showed to have associations with gout and hyperuricaemia in some populations [30, 33].

3.2.10 SLC16A9

The *SLC16A9* gene is located on human chromosome 10q21. The encoded protein has importer activity and monocarboxylic acid transmembrane transporter activity. GWAS studies found gene to have associations with gout and hyperuricaemia in some populations [33, 35].

GWASs also discovered other genes in some populations. These genes were *TRIM46, ACVR2A, LRP2, CNTN4, MUSTN1, SFMBT1, FAM134B, TMEM171, RREB1, VEGFA, SGK1, MLXIPL, PRKAG2, STC1, HNF4G, A1CF, DIP2C, SLC16A9, OVOL1, HNF1A, ACVR1B, ACVRL1, USP2, ATXN2, TSHR, IGF1R, NFAT5, HLF, BCAS3, PRPSAP1, ALDH16A1, ZNF160* [55]. It is likely these genes contribute small portion of risks in the development of hyperuricaemia and gout. Other genes that are responsible for some Mendelian syndromes are also associated with hyperuricaemia and gout. These genes are *HPRT1, PRPS1, G6PC, SLC37A4, AGL, PYGM, PFKM, AMPD1, CPT2, AMPD1, ACADS, ALDOB, UMOD*. These are responsible for the diseases caused congenital errors of purine metabolism, excessive cell death and urate generation and reduced renal excretion of uric acid [26].

3.3 Pharmacogenetics and pharmacogenomics of LUT for gout

The current pharmacogenetics and pharmacogenomics majorly focus on the medications on the three paths that balance the uric acid levels in the serum. Together with treating acute gout, there are about 10 genetic loci that modify the common medications' effectiveness or adverse events in gout management.

3.3.1 The genes that influence xanthine oxidase inhibitors (XOIs)

XOIs are the first line medications in the long-term treatment of hyperuricaemia and gout. Allopurinol and febuxostat are two important XOIs. Allopurinol is transformed into its active metabolite oxypurinol that reversibly blocks xanthine oxidase while febuxostat is a non-purine-selective inhibitor of xanthine oxidase [56]. Allopurinol is a common efficacious ULT but it associates with rare serious adverse drug reactions of Stevens-Johnson syndrome (SJS) and toxic epidermal necrolysis (TEN) [57]. The human leukocyte antigen B allele *HLA-B*5801* was reported to be a genetic marker for allopurinol-induced side effects [58, 59]. Strong associations between *HLA-B*5801* and allopurinol-induced TEN/SJS were found in Hong Kong [60], Korea [61] and Thailand [62]. Genome-wide association study of Stevens-Johnson syndrome and toxic epidermal necrolysis also confirmed that the *HLA-B*5801* allele was associated with allopurinol-induced symptoms in Europe [63]. Patients who are *HLA-B*5801* carriers can be alternatively given febuxostat.

The clinical consideration is the cost of febuxosat as it is much higher than the administration of allopurinol. There is a paucity of evidence about economic value of such testing as allopurinol is an affordable medication. Testing *HLA-B*5801* prior to allopurinol management is cost-effective for Asians and African American, but not for Caucasians or Hispanic in the United States [64]. In Thailand it was also shown highly potential cost-effective intervention [65]. Chinese Han population is a high risk group of the side-effects of allopurinol [14]. In our previous retrospective investigation of *HLA-B*5801* in hyperuricaemia patients in a Han population of China, we found 30 carriers of *HLA-B*5801* allele in 253 cases of hyperuricaemia or gout patients in Chinese Han population (11.9%). Most importantly allopurinol was prescribed in both *HLA-B*5801* positive and negative groups. We also assessed four models with or without genetic screening and management of allopurinol or febuxostat, the results indicated the *HLA-B*5801* screening had significant cost benefit for clinical management for gout patients. The other alleles of HLA locus (for example *HLA-B*1502*) are also responsible for SJS/TEN induced by other drugs [66]. The prevalence of *HLA-B*5801* in hyperuricaemia patients in a Han population of China indicated the importance of genotyping the allele to prevent the severe side-effects induced by allopurinol. *HLA-B*5801* should be screened in all allopurinol-induced TEN patients no matter what their races are. To all SJS/TEN patients, if allopurinol was not administrated, other HLA allele screening should be considered [67, 68]. HLA-DR9 and HLA-DR14 were also found to have associations with the allopurinol induced hypersensitivity in hematologic malignancy [69]. Genetic variation in aldehyde oxidase (AOX1), encoding the enzyme responsible for the conversion of allopurinol to oxypurinol, also was reported to be associated with allopurinol dose and change in serum urate [70]. *ABCG2*, encoding an efflux pump, was associated with SUA reduction and a missense allele (rs2231142) was associated with a reduced response to allopurinol [50].

3.3.2 The genes that influence uricosurics

Uricosurics are the second line of choice to treat hyperuricaemia and gout clinically. Currently three medications are working as uricosurics for renal excretion of uric acid. They are probenecid, benzbromarone (BBR) and lesinurad. BBR and its metabolite 6-hydroxybenzbromarone block the renal reabsorption of uric acid by inhibiting URAT1 in proximal renal tubular cells [11]. BBR undergoes hepatic hydroxylation to 1′-hydroxy BBR and 6-hydroxy BBR. The BBR elimination in serum was affected by genetic polymorphism in drug metabolism [71]. It was demonstrated that CYP2C9 was the main enzyme responsible for the 6-hydroxylation of BBR [72, 73]. *CYP2C9* is highly polymorphic gene and it has around 57 variant alleles [11]. SNP rs1799853 (Cys144Arg) and SNP rs1057910 (Ile359Leu) were the most common poor metabolizer polymorphisms, existing in about 15–22% of Caucasians and 1–9% of Africans. SNP rs1799853 was rare in Asians, while rs1057910 frequencies range from 2 to 11% [74]. rs1799853 could typically results in a 20–30% reduction in maximum velocity (Vmax) for drug substrates whereas rs1057910 can reduce Vmax by as much as 70% [75]. The 144Arg substitution could affect the interaction of CYP2C9 with CYP450 reductase [76], whereas the 359Leu substitution can alters substrate recognition [77]. *CYP2C9*3* homozygotes have significantly reduced clearance of BBR and therefore may be at increased risk of hepatotoxicity [78].

3.3.3 The genes that influence uricase

Rasburicase is an urate oxidase. It is a peroxisomal liver enzyme to catalyze the oxidation of uric acid into the more water-soluble substrates. Urate oxidase is an endogenous enzyme can be found in most mammals but not in humans. The inactivation of the hominoid urate oxidase gene was caused by independent nonsense or frame-shift mutations during evolution [79] . Two nonsense mutations were found in the human urate oxidase gene that makes it non-functional in human [80, 81]. Pegloticase is a recombinant uricase for the treatment of severe, treatment-refractory, chronic gout. It is a third-line treatment for patients who do not tolerate to other treatments [56, 82]. Pegloticase also catalyze uric acid to allantoin which is 5–10 times more soluble than uric acid. Pegloticase is in pegylated form so it can increase its elimination half-life from about 8 hours to 10 or 12 days, and this can decrease the immunogenicity of the foreign uricase protein. Among patients with chronic gout, the use of pegloticase 8 mg either every 2 weeks or every 4 weeks for 6 months resulted in lower uric acid levels compared with placebo [56]. A case of pegloticase-related methemoglobinemia and haemolytic anaemia was reported as it was cause by two mutations in glucose-6-phosphate dehydrogenase (*G6PD*) gene known to confer G6PD deficiency [83]. It was recommended that avoiding the use of rasburicase in patient's homo/hemizygous for G6PD variants that confer deficiency [84].

Loci	Chr	Affecting drug	Uric acid path or gout	Key reference	Pharmaceutical effects
HLA-B5801	6p21	Allopurinol	Uric acid formation, XO inhibitors	[58]	Adverse effect: drug allergic response
HLA-DR9	6p21	Allopurinol	Uric acid formation, XO inhibitors	[69]	Adverse effect: inducing hematologic malignancy
HLA-DR14	6p21	Allopurinol	Uric acid formation, XO inhibitors	[69]	Adverse effect: inducing hematologic malignancy
AOX1	*2q33*	Allopurinol	Uric acid formation, XO inhibitors	[70]	Dose and change in serum urate
ABCG2	*4q22*	Allopurinol	Uric acid formation, XO inhibitors	[50]	Reducing dose response
CYP2C9	10q23	Benzbromarone	Uric acid renal excretion	[71]	Reducing drug clearance and hepatic failure
G6PD	Xq28	Pelgoticase	Uric acid transforming	[83]	Adverse effects: inducing haemolytic anaemia
PTGS2	1q31	NSAID	Acute gout	[86]	Drug response: Aspirin insensitivity
ITGA2	5q11	NSAID	Acute gout	[88]	Drug response: Aspirin insensitivity
ABCB1	7q21	Colchicine	Acute gout	[90]	Drug response

Table 2.
The pharmacogenetic loci that regulating ULT.

3.4 The genes that influence medications for acute gout

Nonsteroidal anti-inflammatory drugs (NSAIDs) are frequently used to quickly relieve the pain and swelling of an acute gout episode and can shorten the attack, but NSAIDs may not be suitable for patients with other comorbidities. A proton pump inhibitor should be offered to people at high risk of NSAID-related gastrointestinal complications [85]. Cyclooxygenase-2 (COX-2) is encoded by prostaglandin-endoperoxide synthase 2 (*PTGS2*). COX-2 catalyzes arachidonic acid to prostaglandin (PG) G2 and H2. A promoter SNP variant of PTGS2-765G>C (rs20417) was shown evidence of association with NSAID response [86, 87]. A recent meta-analysis reported a significant association of the variant with aspirin insensitivity in Chinese population [88]. The variant rs1126643 of integrin subunit alpha 2 gene (*ITGA2*) genetic defects might also increase the risk of having aspirin insensitivity [88]. Colchicine works by decreasing swelling and lessening the build-up of uric acid crystals that cause pain in the affected joint (s). ATP binding cassette subfamily B member 1 (*ABCB1*) gene is highly polymorphic and codes for the drug efflux pump MDR1, and as such is considered an important gene that influences drug metabolisms [89]. The occurrence of colchicine unresponsiveness was significantly higher in patients who were homozygous or heterozygous for the major allele (*ABCB1* 3435C) than in minor allele homozygotes [90]. To date, there is no information on whether these polymorphisms are associated with nonresponse in patients with gout.

The potential pharmacological loci for hyperuricaemia and gout were listed in **Table 2**.

4. Epigenetic factors and environmental factors for hyperuricaemia and gout

4.1 DNA methylation

GAWs have identified dozens of loci associated with gout, but for most cases, the risk genes and the underlying molecular mechanisms contributing to these associations are unknown. Epigenetics studies investigate heritable change in gene expression caused by molecules that bind to DNA without change the actual DNA sequence. There are three main classes of epigenetic marks as DNA methylation, modification of histone tails and noncoding RNAs. DNA methylation has been found to associate with many complicated diseases. Hypomethylation at the promoter region of the gout-risk gene *NRBP1* can lead to enhanced gene expression both in vitro and in vivo, contributing to the development of gout [91]. Chinese Han population with gout had a significant association between *CCL2* promoter hypomethylation and the risk of the disease [92]. Hypermethylation of uromodolin (UMOD) observed in gout patients might reduce the gene expression, leading to an augmented risk of gout [93]. A research on genetic variations in the DNA methyltransferases (DNMTs) gene identified *DNMT1* SNP rs2228611 polymorphism may be involved in the pathogenesis of gout [94].

4.2 miRNA

MicroRNAs (miRNAs) are non-coding RNA species that are highly evolutionarily conserved in human. Up to 5000 miRNAs were identified in human cells. miRNAs are key regulators of the expression of numerous targets at the post-transcriptional level [95]. They are implicated in various cell processes including cell differentiation, metabolism, and inflammation. Experimental evidence suggests that metabolic deregulation is a commonality between these different pathological entities, and that miRNAs are key players in the modulation of metabolic routes [96]. Recent studies have shown that interleukin (IL)-1β is a key inflammatory mediator in acute gouty arthritis (GA), and its level is regulated by miRNAs. Five miRNAs (hsa-miR-30c-1-3p, hsa-miR-488-3p, hsa-miR-550a-3p, hsa-miR-663a, and hsa-miR-920) were found to possibly target IL-1β. MSU crystals in GA patient could inhibit expression of miR-488 and miR-920 and the two miRNAs could directly target the 3′-UTR of IL-1β [97]. MSU crystal-induced IL-1 secretion can be targeted for the new therapeutic strategies in the treatment of acute gout [98].

4.3 Exosomes

Exosomes are best defined as extracellular vesicles that are released from cells upon fusion of an intermediate endocytic compartment, the multivesicular body (MVB), with the plasma membrane. Exosomes can be produced by most cell types. Exosomes derived from immunosuppressive dendritic cells (DCs) have been found to confer potent and lasting immunosuppressive effects, similar to their parental DC [99, 100]. Their protein content largely reflects that of the parental cells and is enriched in certain molecules including adhesion molecules, membrane trafficking molecules, cytoskeleton molecules, heat-shock proteins, cytoplasmic enzymes, signal transduction proteins, and cell-specific antigens [101–103]. Exosomes also contain functional mRNA and microRNAs molecules [104]. Certain types of exosomes have been shown to confer immunosuppressive effects in different disease models including RA and gout. It is likely that exosomes represent a novel effective and safe therapeutic approach for treating arthritis [105]. In a neutrophil-derived microvesicles (PMN-Ecto) studied for a murine model of MSU-induced. PMN-Ecto from joint aspirates of patients with gouty arthritis had similar anti-inflammatory properties [106]. In a study for investigating the effects of MSU on synovial fibroblasts to elucidate the process of MSU-mediated synovial inflammation, human synovial fibroblasts were stimulated with MSU in the presence or absence of serum amyloid A [107]. MSU stimulation resulted in the activation of caspase-1 and production of active IL-1β and IL-1α. These findings provide insight into the molecular processes underlying the synovial inflammatory condition of gout [108].

4.4 Microbiota

The human microbiota consists of the 10–100 trillion symbiotic microbial cells in each person including primarily bacteria in the gut. The human microbiome refers the genes these cells harbor [109]. Microbiota was found to play the important roles for the development of personalized medicine. Whole microbial genome sequencing revealed the extraordinary diversity of microorganisms and their vast genetic and metabolic repertoire [110]. In a cohort study with 33 healthy and 35 gout patients, the intestinal microbiota of patients were highly distinct from healthy individuals in both organismal and functional structures. In gout, there were more Bacteroides caccae and Bacteroides xylanisolvens, there were less or absence Faecalibacterium prausnitzii and Bifidobacterium pseudocatenulatum. Intestinal microbiota of gout is more similar to those of type-2 diabetes than to liver cirrhosis, whereas depletion of Faecalibacterium prausnitzii and reduced butyrate biosynthesis were shared in each of the metabolic syndromes [111].

4.5 Metabolites

Metabolites are the intermediate products of metabolic reactions catalyzed by various enzymes that naturally occur within cells and play vital roles in cell growth, differentials and proliferations. In a study analyzing 355 metabolites in 1764 individuals and constructed a metabolite network around serum urate. The effect of sex and urate lowering medication on all 38 metabolites assigned to the three network. The three network included the well-known pathway of purine metabolism, as well as several dipeptides, a group of essential amino acids, and a group of steroids. Of the 38 assigned metabolites, 25 showed strong differences between sexes. The findings highlight pathways that are important in the regulation of serum urate and suggest that dipeptides, amino acids, and steroid hormones are playing a role in its regulation [112].

4.6 The relationships between genetic factors and environmental factors for hyperuricaemia and gout

The genetic influence and environmental factors should be considered equally importance for hyperuricaemia and gout. Determining the extent to which environmental versus genetic factors are responsible for particular phenotypes such as gout or hyperuricaemia is a central question in gout or hyperuricaemia research. Elucidating associations between genotype and phenotype has been a central goal in human health research for some time [113]. The complications in cellular process of hyperuricaemia mean many genes may have interactions with each other for the regulation of the products of uric acid in cells; they may not be identifiable even in approaches with GWASs. The environmental factors can also interact with genetic factors that make the process even more complicated. For clinicians, it is important to understand the etiological causes for complicate diseases and always consider both genetic and environmental factors play important roles in hyperuricaemia and gout.

5. Personalized medicine for ULT and gout

The personalized medicine aims to provide the right treatments in the right time for individual patients with hyperuricaemia and gout. The genetics variants that underlie diseases and influence the medications will play great roles for the management of gout in near future. Therapeutics best suited for an individual's genotype genetic origins of disease and drug response for LUT including adverse events. Precision medicine has made great progress due to the rapid development of pharmacogenomics research. Clinically, patients' age, race, and gender are all associated with epigenetic status [114]. Together with the developments of miRNA profiling, epigenetics investigation, metabolites screening and microbiota research it will make personalized medicine possible for gout management.

5.1 Intrinsic factor assessment

For intrinsic factor assessment, patients age, gender, geographic residence, social economic status and other conditions for heart, kidney and liver, allergic status are all important factors to be considered for clinical managements of hyperuricaemia and gout. These factors should be considered to decide the medication choice, the dosage of medications. The decision should be managed to benefit for individual patients with hyperuricaemia and gout.

5.2 The life style assessment

In clinical practice, lifestyle changes are frequently urged for prevention and management of gout [115]. It is advocated to promote healthy eating and drinking for gout patients, such as reducing intake of beer, sugar-sweetened drinks, and purine-rich foods such as meat, offal and seafood. Increased intake of cherries, omega-3 fatty acids, low fat milk and coffee are also advocated [116]. There was evidence for a non-additive interaction of sugar-sweetened drinks consumption with a urate-associated variant of *SLC2A9* for the risk of gout [117] . Alcohol intake with T allele of lipoprotein receptor-related protein 2 gene (*LRP2*) rs2544390 was reported in determining the risk of hyperuricaemia and gout [118, 119].

5.3 The genetic inheritance and epigenetic affect

The studies of genetic inheritance of gout and hyperuricaemia provide a lot useful information. More than 40 genetic loci only can explain less than 10% of high uric acid levels in serum. We also need to consider the genetic background in different ethnical populations. The further efforts will be to understand the functional roles of the novel genes in the pathways of uric acid metabolism. The investigation can identify the new pharmacological target for gout and bring new therapeutic tools from preventing to treating gout patients [55]. miRNAs and epigenetic screening are also helpful to identify the regulator elements for potential gout gene's expression.

5.4 Microbiome and metabolite factors

Microbiome and metabolite factors are also need to be considered when managing gout patients clinically. At the present times, not enough reports have been published in the field. It can be useful to exam the intestinal levels of Bacteroides caccae, Bacteroides xylanisolvens, Faecalibacterium prausnitzii, Bifidobacterium pseudocatenulatum in gout patients. Screening key metabolites in serum may also helpful in clinical management of gout and hyperuricaemia patients.

5.5 The pharmacogenetic consideration

Total about 10 genetic loci were identified to influence the medications of gout. These loci can be used to predict the drug's response and adverse effects. For

Assessments	Considering factors
Intrinsic factor assessment	Age; gender; geographic residence; other conditions for heart, kidney and liver, allergic history etc
Life style assessment	Diet and activities; the in-taking of food with rich purines—such as meat, poultry, and seafood; alcohol consumption etc
Genetic inheritance	Suspected gene screening such as *SLC2A9, ABCG2, GCKR*, *PDZK1* and other SLC loci etc.
Epigenetic factors	miRNA; methylation screening for suspected loci; histone methylation etc
Environmental factors	Microbiota; metabolites screening
Pharmacogenetics consideration	For NSAIDs, screening *PTGS2, ABCG2;* for colchicine, screening *ABCB1;* for XO inhibitor allopurinol, screening *HLA-B5801, HLA-DR9, HLA-DR14, AOX1* and *ABCG2;* for Benzbromarone, screening *CYP2C9; for* Pelgoticase, screening *G6PD*

Table 3.
Personalized medicine approaches for management of LUT for gout.

treating acute gout with NSAIDs, *PTGS2, ABCG2* should be screened as the variants affect aspirin sensitivity. For colchicine treatment, *ABCB1* should be screened as the variant affect drug's response; For XO inhibitor allopurinol, *HLA-B5801, HLA-DR9*, *HLA-DR14*, *AOX1*and *ABCG2* should be screened as the variants may induce adverse events or response changes. For benzbromarone, *CYP2C9* should be screened as the variant may affect drug clearance and cause side effects. For pegloticase, *G6PD* should be screened as the variant may have adverse effects to induce haemolytic anaemia.

The personalized factors have been summarized in **Table 3**.

6. Summary

Personalized medicine has made great progress due to the development of the technology in genetic and genomic approaches. The ultimate goal for personal medicine of gout management is to provide the best medical advice and best medical treatment according to conditions of individual patients. The patient conditions including age, gender, ethnic group, life styles, genetic variations for common gout associated genes are important factors for clinical managements. Most importantly the pharmacogenetic loci for the common medications for gout provide useful guidance for individual patients. The developments of miRNA profiling, epigenetics investigation, metabolites screening and microbiota research will make personalized medicine even more in great details for management. It will revolutionize medical cares for gout patients in near future.

Acknowledgements

Dewen Yan is supported by National Natural Science Foundation of China. Youming Zhang is supported by Asmarley Foundation in the UK.

Abbreviations

ABC	ATP-binding cassette
ABCB1	ATP binding cassette subfamily B member 1
ABCG2	ATP binding cassette, subfamily G, member 2
ADRB3	adrenergic receptor beta-3
AHS	allopurinol hypersensitivity syndrome
BBR	benzbromarone
CCA4	congenital cerulean cataract 4
COX2	cyclooxygenase-2
CNV	copy number variant
DCs	dendritic cells
DNMTs	DNA methyltransferases
EC	endothelial cell
GA	gouty arthritis
GCKR	glucokinase regulator
GWAS	genome-wide association study
G6PD	glucose-6-phosphate dehydrogenase
HDL	high-density lipoproteins
hnRNPs	heteregeneous ribonucleoproteins
HNF4G	hepatocyte nuclear factor 4 gamma

HNF4A	hepatocyte nuclear factor 4 alpha
HLA	human leukocyte antigen
INDEL	insertion and deletion of short segments of DNA
ITGA2	integrin subunit alpha 2
LRP2	lipoprotein receptor-related protein 2
miRNA	micro RNA
MODY	maturity-onset diabetes of the young
MSU	monosodium urate
MVB	multivesicular body
NSAIDs	nonsteroid anti-inflammatory drugs
PAK	p21-activated protein kinase
PTGS2	prostaglandin-endoperoxide synthase 2
SAA	serum amyloid A
SCAR	serious cutaneous adverse reactions
SNPs	single nuclear polymorphisms
siRNA	small interfering RNA
SJS	Stevens-Johnson syndrome
SU	serum urate
SUA	serum uric acid
TEN	toxic epidermal necrolysis
TGF	transforming growth factor
ULT	urate-lowering therapy
UMOD	uromodolin
Vmax	maximum velocity
VNTRs	variable number of tandem repeats
XOI	xanthine oxidase inhibitor

Author details

Dewen Yan[1*] and Youming Zhang[2*]

1 Department of Endocrinology, Xiangya-Shenzhen Endocrinology and Metabolism Center, The First Affiliated Hospital of Shenzhen University, Shenzhen, PR China

2 Functional Genomics Group, Genomic Medicine Section, National Heart and Lung Institute, Imperial College London, UK

*Address all correspondence to: y.zhang@imperial.ac.uk and yandw963@126.com

References

[1] Pillinger MH, Rosenthal P, Abeles AM. Hyperuricemia and gout: New insights into pathogenesis and treatment. Bulletin of the NYU Hospital for Joint Diseases. 2007;**65**(3):215-221

[2] Chen LX, Schumacher HR. Gout: An evidence-based review. Journal of Clinical Rheumatology: Practical Reports on Rheumatic & Musculoskeletal Diseases. 2008;**14** (5 Suppl):S55-S62

[3] Smith E, Hoy D, Cross M, Merriman TR, Vos T, Buchbinder R, et al. The global burden of gout: Estimates from the global burden of disease 2010 study. Annals of the Rheumatic Diseases. 2014;**73**(8):1470-1476

[4] Ragab G, Elshahaly M, Bardin T. Gout: An old disease in new perspective—A review. Journal of Advanced Research. 2017;**8**(5):495-511

[5] Kuo CF, Grainge MJ, Zhang W, Doherty M. Global epidemiology of gout: Prevalence, incidence and risk factors. Nature Reviews Rheumatology. 2015;**11**(11):649-662

[6] Kiadaliri AA, Uhlig T, Englund M. Burden of gout in the Nordic region, 1990-2015: Findings from the global burden of disease study 2015. Scandinavian Journal of Rheumatology. 2018;**47**(5):410-417

[7] Liu R, Han C, Wu D, Xia X, Gu J, Guan H, et al. Prevalence of hyperuricemia and gout in mainland China from 2000 to 2014: A systematic review and meta-analysis. BioMed Research International. 2015;**2015**:762820

[8] Maiuolo J, Oppedisano F, Gratteri S, Muscoli C, Mollace V. Regulation of uric acid metabolism and excretion. International Journal of Cardiology. 2016;**213**:8-14

[9] Palmer TM, Nordestgaard BG, Benn M, Tybjaerg-Hansen A, Davey Smith G, Lawlor DA, et al. Association of plasma uric acid with ischaemic heart disease and blood pressure: Mendelian randomisation analysis of two large cohorts. BMJ. 2013;**347**:f4262

[10] Hughes K, Flynn T, de Zoysa J, Dalbeth N, Merriman TR. Mendelian randomization analysis associates increased serum urate, due to genetic variation in uric acid transporters, with improved renal function. Kidney International. 2014;**85**(2):344-351

[11] Roberts RL, Stamp LK. Pharmacogenetic considerations in the treatment of gout. Pharmacogenomics. 2015;**16**(6):619-629

[12] Bannasch D, Safra N, Young A, Karmi N, Schaible RS, Ling GV. Mutations in the SLC2A9 gene cause hyperuricosuria and hyperuricemia in the dog. PLoS Genetics. 2008;**4**(11):e1000246

[13] Drug, Therapeutics B. Latest guidance on the management of gout. BMJ. 2018;**362**:k2893

[14] Khanna D, Fitzgerald JD, Khanna PP, Bae S, Singh MK, Neogi T, et al. 2012 American College of Rheumatology guidelines for management of gout. Part 1: Systematic nonpharmacologic and pharmacologic therapeutic approaches to hyperuricemia. Arthritis Care & Research. 2012;**64**(10):1431-1446

[15] Zhang W, Doherty M, Bardin T, Pascual E, Barskova V, Conaghan P, et al. EULAR evidence based recommendations for gout. Part II: Management. Report of a task force of the EULAR Standing Committee for International Clinical Studies Including Therapeutics (ESCISIT). Annals of the Rheumatic Diseases. 2006;**65**(10):1312-1324

[16] Motulsky AG. Drug reactions enzymes, and biochemical genetics. Journal of the American Medical Association. 1957;**165**(7):835-837

[17] Weinshilboum R. Inheritance and drug response. The New England Journal of Medicine. 2003;**348**(6):529-537

[18] Evans WE, McLeod HL. Pharmacogenomics-drug disposition, drug targets, and side effects. The New England Journal of Medicine. 2003;**348**(6):538-549

[19] Genomes Project C, Auton A, Brooks LD, Durbin RM, Garrison EP, Kang HM, et al. A global reference for human genetic variation. Nature. 2015;**526**(7571):68-74

[20] Mills RE, Luttig CT, Larkins CE, Beauchamp A, Tsui C, Pittard WS, et al. An initial map of insertion and deletion (INDEL) variation in the human genome. Genome Research. 2006;**16**(9):1182-1190

[21] Rigat B, Hubert C, Alhenc-Gelas F, Cambien F, Corvol P, Soubrier F. An insertion/deletion polymorphism in the angiotensin I-converting enzyme gene accounting for half the variance of serum enzyme levels. The Journal of Clinical Investigation. 1990;**86**(4):1343-1346

[22] Cook EH Jr, Scherer SW. Copy-number variations associated with neuropsychiatric conditions. Nature. 2008;**455**(7215):919-923

[23] Zhang Y, Moffatt MF, Cookson WO. Genetic and genomic approaches to asthma: New insights for the origins. Current Opinion in Pulmonary Medicine. 2012;**18**(1):6-13

[24] Welter D, Mac Arthur J, Morales J, Burdett T, Hall P, Junkins H, et al. The NHGRI GWAS Catalog, a curated resource of SNP-trait associations. Nucleic Acids Research. 2014;**42**(Database issue):D1001-D1006

[25] Dehghan A, Kottgen A, Yang Q, Hwang SJ, Kao WL, Rivadeneira F, et al. Association of three genetic loci with uric acid concentration and risk of gout: A genome-wide association study. Lancet. 2008;**372**(9654):1953-1961

[26] Reginato AM, Mount DB, Yang I, Choi HK. The genetics of hyperuricaemia and gout. Nature Reviews Rheumatology. 2012;**8**(10):610-621

[27] Charles BA, Shriner D, Doumatey A, Chen G, Zhou J, Huang H, et al. A genome-wide association study of serum uric acid in African Americans. BMC Medical Genomics. 2011;**4**:17

[28] Tin A, Woodward OM, Kao WH, Liu CT, Lu X, Nalls MA, et al. Genome-wide association study for serum urate concentrations and gout among African Americans identifies genomic risk loci and a novel URAT1 loss-of-function allele. Human Molecular Genetics. 2011;**20**(20):4056-4068

[29] Kamatani Y, Matsuda K, Okada Y, Kubo M, Hosono N, Daigo Y, et al. Genome-wide association study of hematological and biochemical traits in a Japanese population. Nature Genetics. 2010;**42**(3):210-215

[30] Okada Y, Sim X, Go MJ, Wu JY, Gu D, Takeuchi F, et al. Meta-analysis identifies multiple loci associated with kidney function-related traits in east Asian populations. Nature Genetics. 2012;**44**(8):904-909

[31] Doring A, Gieger C, Mehta D, Gohlke H, Prokisch H, Coassin S, et al. SLC2A9 influences uric acid concentrations with pronounced sex-specific effects. Nature Genetics. 2008;**40**(4):430-436

[32] Karns R, Zhang G, Sun G, Rao Indugula S, Cheng H, Havas-Augustin D,

et al. Genome-wide association of serum uric acid concentration: Replication of sequence variants in an island population of the Adriatic coast of Croatia. Annals of Human Genetics. 2012;**76**(2):121-127

[33] Kottgen A, Albrecht E, Teumer A, Vitart V, Krumsiek J, Hundertmark C, et al. Genome-wide association analyses identify 18 new loci associated with serum urate concentrations. Nature Genetics. 2013;**45**(2):145-154

[34] Wallace C, Newhouse SJ, Braund P, Zhang F, Tobin M, Falchi M, et al. Genome-wide association study identifies genes for biomarkers of cardiovascular disease: Serum urate and dyslipidemia. The American Journal of Human Genetics. 2008;**82**(1):139-149

[35] Kolz M, Johnson T, Sanna S, Teumer A, Vitart V, Perola M, et al. Meta-analysis of 28, 141 individuals identifies common variants within five new loci that influence uric acid concentrations. PLoS Genetics. 2009;**5**(6):e1000504

[36] Sulem P, Gudbjartsson DF, Walters GB, Helgadottir HT, Helgason A, Gudjonsson SA, et al. Identification of low-frequency variants associated with gout and serum uric acid levels. Nature Genetics. 2011;**43**(11):1127-1130

[37] Vitart V, Rudan I, Hayward C, Gray NK, Floyd J, Palmer CN, et al. SLC2A9 is a newly identified urate transporter influencing serum urate concentration, urate excretion and gout. Nature Genetics. 2008;**40**(4):437-442

[38] McArdle PF, Parsa A, Chang YP, Weir MR, O'Connell JR, Mitchell BD, et al. Association of a common nonsynonymous variant in GLUT9 with serum uric acid levels in old order amish. Arthritis and Rheumatism. 2008;**58**(9):2874-2881

[39] Li S, Sanna S, Maschio A, Busonero F, Usala G, Mulas A, et al. The GLUT9 gene is associated with serum uric acid levels in sardinia and chianti cohorts. PLoS Genetics. 2007;**3**(11):e194

[40] Stark K, Reinhard W, Neureuther K, Wiedmann S, Sedlacek K, Baessler A, et al. Association of common polymorphisms in GLUT9 gene with gout but not with coronary artery disease in a large case-control study. PLoS One. 2008;**3**(4):e1948

[41] DeBosch BJ, Kluth O, Fujiwara H, Schurmann A, Moley K. Early-onset metabolic syndrome in mice lacking the intestinal uric acid transporter SLC2A9. Nature Communications. 2014;**5**:4642

[42] Auberson M, Stadelmann S, Stoudmann C, Seuwen K, Koesters R, Thorens B, et al. SLC2A9 (GLUT9) mediates urate reabsorption in the mouse kidney. Pflügers Archiv: European Journal of Physiology. 2018;**470**(12):1739-1751

[43] Itahana Y, Han R, Barbier S, Lei Z, Rozen S, Itahana K. The uric acid transporter SLC2A9 is a direct target gene of the tumor suppressor p 53 contributing to antioxidant defense. Oncogene. 2015;**34**(14):1799-1810

[44] Augustin R, Carayannopoulos MO, Dowd LO, Phay JE, Moley JF, Moley KH. Identification and characterization of human glucose transporter-like protein-9 (GLUT9): Alternative splicing alters trafficking. The Journal of Biological Chemistry. 2004;**279**(16):16229-16236

[45] Yang Q, Kottgen A, Dehghan A, Smith AV, Glazer NL, Chen MH, et al. Multiple genetic loci influence serum urate levels and their relationship with gout and cardiovascular disease risk factors. Circulation. Cardiovascular Genetics. 2010;**3**(6):523-530

[46] Campbell PK, Zong Y, Yang S, Zhou S, Rubnitz JE, Sorrentino BP. Identification of a novel, tissue-specific ABCG2 promoter expressed in pediatric acute megakaryoblastic

leukemia. Leukemia Research. 2011;**35**(10):1321-1329

[47] Huls M, Brown CD, Windass AS, Sayer R, van den Heuvel JJ, Heemskerk S, et al. The breast cancer resistance protein transporter ABCG2 is expressed in the human kidney proximal tubule apical membrane. Kidney International. 2008;**73**(2):220-225

[48] Merriman T. Genomic influences on hyperuricemia and gout. Rheumatic Diseases Clinics of North America. 2017;**43**(3):389-399

[49] Chen CJ, Tseng CC, Yen JH, Chang JG, Chou WC, Chu HW, et al. ABCG2 contributes to the development of gout and hyperuricemia in a genome-wide association study. Scientific Reports. 2018;**8**(1):3137

[50] Wen CC, Yee SW, Liang X, Hoffmann TJ, Kvale MN, Banda Y, et al. Genome-wide association study identifies ABCG2 (BCRP) as an allopurinol transporter and a determinant of drug response. Clinical Pharmacology and Therapeutics. 2015;**97**(5):518-525

[51] Uchino H, Tamai I, Yamashita K, Minemoto Y, Sai Y, Yabuuchi H, et al. p-Aminohippuric acid transport at renal apical membrane mediated by human inorganic phosphate transporter NPT1. Biochemical and Biophysical Research Communications. 2000;**270**(1):254-259

[52] Riches PL, Wright AF, Ralston SH. Recent insights into the pathogenesis of hyperuricaemia and gout. Human Molecular Genetics. 2009;**18**(R2):R177-R184

[53] Tin A, Li Y, Brody JA, Nutile T, Chu AY, Huffman JE, et al. Large-scale whole-exome sequencing association studies identify rare functional variants influencing serum urate levels. Nature Communications. 2018;**9**(1):4228

[54] Ketharnathan S, Leask M, Boocock J, Phipps-Green AJ, Antony J, O'Sullivan JM, et al. A non-coding genetic variant maximally associated with serum urate levels is functionally linked to HNF4A-dependent PDZK1 expression. Human Molecular Genetics. 2018;**27**(22):3964-3973

[55] Major TJ, Dalbeth N, Stahl EA, Merriman TR. An update on the genetics of hyperuricaemia and gout. Nature Reviews Rheumatology. 2018;**14**(6):341-353

[56] Sundy JS, Baraf HS, Yood RA, Edwards NL, Gutierrez-Urena SR, Treadwell EL, et al. Efficacy and tolerability of pegloticase for the treatment of chronic gout in patients refractory to conventional treatment: Two randomized controlled trials. Journal of the American Medical Association. 2011;**306**(7):711-720

[57] Roujeau JC, Kelly JP, Naldi L, Rzany B, Stern RS, Anderson T, et al. Medication use and the risk of Stevens-Johnson syndrome or toxic epidermal necrolysis. The New England Journal of Medicine. 1995;**333**(24):1600-1607

[58] Hung SI, Chung WH, Liou LB, Chu CC, Lin M, Huang HP, et al. HLA-B*5801 allele as a genetic marker for severe cutaneous adverse reactions caused by allopurinol. Proceedings of the National Academy of Sciences of the United States of America. 2005;**102**(11):4134-4139

[59] Somkrua R, Eickman EE, Saokaew S, Lohitnavy M, Chaiyakunapruk N. Association of HLA-B*5801 allele and allopurinol-induced Stevens Johnson syndrome and toxic epidermal necrolysis: A systematic review and meta-analysis. BMC Medical Genetics. 2011;**12**:118

[60] Chiu ML, Hu M, Ng MH, Yeung CK, Chan JC, Chang MM, et al. Association between HLA-B*58: 01 allele and

severe cutaneous adverse reactions with allopurinol in Han Chinese in Hong Kong. The British Journal of Dermatology. 2012;**167**(1):44-49

[61] Kang HR, Jee YK, Kim YS, Lee CH, Jung JW, Kim SH, et al. Positive and negative associations of HLA class I alleles with allopurinol-induced SCARs in Koreans. Pharmacogenetics and Genomics. 2011;**21**(5):303-307

[62] Tassaneeyakul W, Jantararoungtong T, Chen P, Lin PY, Tiamkao S, Khunarkornsiri U, et al. Strong association between HLA-B*5801 and allopurinol-induced Stevens-Johnson syndrome and toxic epidermal necrolysis in a Thai population. Pharmacogenetics and Genomics. 2009;**19**(9):704-709

[63] Genin E, Schumacher M, Roujeau JC, Naldi L, Liss Y, Kazma R, et al. Genome-wide association study of Stevens-Johnson syndrome and toxic epidermal necrolysis in Europe. Orphanet Journal of Rare Diseases. 2011;**6**:52

[64] Jutkowitz E, Dubreuil M, Lu N, Kuntz KM, Choi HK. The cost-effectiveness of HLA-B*5801 screening to guide initial urate-lowering therapy for gout in the United States. Seminars in Arthritis and Rheumatism. 2017;**46**(5):594-600

[65] Saokaew S, Tassaneeyakul W, Maenthaisong R, Chaiyakunapruk N. Cost-effectiveness analysis of HLA-B*5801 testing in preventing allopurinol-induced SJS/TEN in Thai population. PloS One. 2014;**9**(4):e94294

[66] Dodiuk-Gad RP, Chung WH, Valeyrie-Allanore L, Shear NH. Stevens-Johnson syndrome and toxic epidermal necrolysis: An update. American Journal of Clinical Dermatology. 2015;**16**(6):475-493

[67] Cheng H, Yan D, Zuo X, Liu J, Liu W, Zhang Y. A retrospective investigation of HLA-B*5801 in hyperuricemia patients in a Han population of China. Pharmacogenetics and Genomics. 2018;**28**(5):117-124

[68] Yan D, Zhang Y. A response letter to allopurinol-induced toxic epidermal necrolysis and association with HLA-B*5801 in white patients. Pharmacogenetics and Genomics. 2018;**28**(12):268-269

[69] Jung JW, Kim JY, Yoon SS, Cho SH, Park SY, Kang HR. HLA-DR9 and DR14 are associated with the allopurinol-induced hypersensitivity in hematologic malignancy. The Tohoku Journal of Experimental Medicine. 2014;**233**(2):95-102

[70] Carroll MB, Smith DM, Shaak TL. Genomic sequencing of uric acid metabolizing and clearing genes in relationship to xanthine oxidase inhibitor dose. Rheumatology International. 2017;**37**(3):445-453

[71] Walter-Sack I, Gresser U, Adjan M, Kamilli I, Ittensohn A, de Vries JX, et al. Variation of benzbromarone elimination in man—A population study. European Journal of Clinical Pharmacology. 1990;**39**(2):173-176

[72] McDonald MG, Rettie AE. Sequential metabolism and bioactivation of the hepatotoxin benzbromarone: Formation of glutathione adducts from a catechol intermediate. Chemical Research in Toxicology. 2007;**20**(12):1833-1842

[73] Kobayashi K, Kajiwara E, Ishikawa M, Oka H, Chiba K. Identification of CYP isozymes involved in benzbromarone metabolism in human liver microsomes. Biopharmaceutics & Drug Disposition. 2012;**33**(8):466-473

[74] Zhou SF, Zhou ZW, Huang M. Polymorphisms of human cytochrome P 450 2C9 and the functional relevance. Toxicology. 2010;**278**(2):165-188

[75] Wei L, Locuson CW, Tracy TS. Polymorphic variants of CYP2C9: Mechanisms involved in reduced catalytic activity. Molecular Pharmacology. 2007;**72**(5):1280-1288

[76] Crespi CL, Miller VP. The R144C change in the CYP2C9*2 allele alters interaction of the cytochrome P 450 with NADPH: Cytochrome P 450 oxidoreductase. Pharmacogenetics. 1997;7(3):203-210

[77] Gotoh O. Substrate recognition sites in cytochrome P 450 family 2 (CYP2) proteins inferred from comparative analyses of amino acid and coding nucleotide sequences. The Journal of Biological Chemistry. 1992;**267**(1):83-90

[78] Uchida S, Shimada K, Misaka S, Imai H, Katoh Y, Inui N, et al. Benzbromarone pharmacokinetics and pharmacodynamics in different cytochrome P 450 2C9 genotypes. Drug Metabolism and Pharmacokinetics. 2010;**25**(6):605-610

[79] Oda M, Satta Y, Takenaka O, Takahata N. Loss of urate oxidase activity in hominoids and its evolutionary implications. Molecular Biology and Evolution. 2002;**19**(5):640-653

[80] Wu XW, Lee CC, Muzny DM, Caskey CT. Urate oxidase: Primary structure and evolutionary implications. Proceedings of the National Academy of Sciences of the United States of America. 1989;**86**(23):9412-9416

[81] Wu XW, Muzny DM, Lee CC, Caskey CT. Two independent mutational events in the loss of urate oxidase during hominoid evolution. Journal of Molecular Evolution. 1992;**34**(1):78-84

[82] Dalbeth N, Merriman TR, Stamp LK. Gout: The Lancet. 2016;**388**(10055): 2039-2052

[83] Geraldino-Pardilla L, Sung D, Xu JZ, Shirazi M, Hod EA, Francis RO. Methaemoglobinaemia and haemolysis following pegloticase infusion for refractory gout in a patient with a falsely negative glucose-6-phosphate dehydrogenase deficiency result. Rheumatology. 2014;**53**(12):2310-2311

[84] McDonagh EM, Thorn CF, Callaghan JT, Altman RB, Klein TE. Pharm GKB summary: Uric acid-lowering drugs pathway, pharmacodynamics. Pharmacogenetics and Genomics. 2014;**24**(9):464-476

[85] Richette P, Doherty M, Pascual E, Barskova V, Becce F, Castaneda-Sanabria J, et al. 2016 updated EULAR evidence-based recommendations for the management of gout. Annals of the Rheumatic Diseases. 2017;**76**(1):29-42

[86] Thorn CF, Grosser T, Klein TE, Altman RB. Pharm GKB summary: Very important pharmacogene information for PTGS2. Pharmacogenetics and Genomics. 2011;**21**(9):607-613

[87] Skarke C, Schuss P, Kirchhof A, Doehring A, Geisslinger G, Lotsch J. Pyrosequencing of polymorphisms in the COX-2 gene (PTGS2) with reported clinical relevance. Pharmacogenomics. 2007;**8**(12):1643-1660

[88] Weng Z, Li X, Li Y, Lin J, Peng F, Niu W. The association of four common polymorphisms from four candidate genes (COX-1, COX-2, ITGA2B, ITGA2) with aspirin insensitivity: A meta-analysis. PloS One. 2013;**8**(11):e78093

[89] Hodges LM, Markova SM, Chinn LW, Gow JM, Kroetz DL, Klein TE, et al. Very important pharmacogene summary: ABCB1 (MDR1, P-glycoprotein). Pharmacogenetics and Genomics. 2011;**21**(3):152-161

[90] Tufan A, Babaoglu MO, Akdogan A, Yasar U, Calguneri M, Kalyoncu U, et al. Association of drug transporter gene

ABCB1 (MDR1) 3435C to T polymorphism with colchicine response in familial Mediterranean fever. The Journal of Rheumatology. 2007;**34**(7):1540-1544

[91] Zhu Z, Meng W, Liu P, Zhu X, Liu Y, Zou H. DNA hypomethylation of a transcription factor binding site within the promoter of a gout risk gene NRBP1 upregulates its expression by inhibition of TFAP2A binding. Clinical Epigenetics. 2017;**9**:99

[92] Li B, Chen X, Jiang Y, Yang Y, Zhong J, Zhou C, et al. CCL2 promoter hypomethylation is associated with gout risk in Chinese Han male population. Immunology Letters. 2017;**190**:15-19

[93] Yang Y, Chen X, Hu H, Jiang Y, Yu H, Dai J, et al. Elevated UMOD methylation level in peripheral blood is associated with gout risk. Scientific Reports. 2017;**7**(1):11196

[94] Zhong X, Peng Y, Yao C, Qing Y, Yang Q, Guo X, et al. Association of DNA methyltransferase polymorphisms with susceptibility to primary gouty arthritis. Biomedical Reports. 2016;**5**(4):467-472

[95] Londin E, Loher P, Telonis AG, Quann K, Clark P, Jing Y, et al. Analysis of 13 cell types reveals evidence for the expression of numerous novel primate- and tissue-specific micro RNAs. Proceedings of the National Academy of Sciences of the United States of America. 2015;**112**(10):E1106-E1115

[96] Papanagnou P, Stivarou T, Tsironi M. The role of mi RNAs in common inflammatory arthropathies: Osteoarthritis and gouty arthritis. Biomolecules. 2016;**6**(4):44

[97] Zhou W, Wang Y, Wu R, He Y, Su Q, Shi G. Micro RNA-488 and -920 regulate the production of proinflammatory cytokines in acute gouty arthritis. Arthritis Research & Therapy. 2017;**19**(1):203

[98] So A, Dumusc A, Nasi S. The role of IL-1 in gout: From bench to bedside. Rheumatology. 2018;**57**(suppl_1):i12-i19

[99] Morelli AE, Larregina AT, Shufesky WJ, Sullivan ML, Stolz DB, Papworth GD, et al. Endocytosis, intracellular sorting, and processing of exosomes by dendritic cells. Blood. 2004;**104**(10):3257-3266

[100] Denzer K, Kleijmeer MJ, Heijnen HF, Stoorvogel W, Geuze HJ. Exosome: From internal vesicle of the multivesicular body to intercellular signaling device. Journal of Cell Science. 2000;**113**(Pt 19):3365-3374

[101] Thery C, Zitvogel L, Amigorena S. Exosomes: Composition, biogenesis and function. Nature Reviews Immunology. 2002;**2**(8):569-579

[102] Thery C, Ostrowski M, Segura E. Membrane vesicles as conveyors of immune responses. Nature Reviews Immunology. 2009;**9**(8):581-593

[103] Matsuo H, Chevallier J, Mayran N, Le Blanc I, Ferguson C, Faure J, et al. Role of LBPA and Alix in multivesicular liposome formation and endosome organization. Science. 2004;**303**(5657):531-534

[104] Valadi H, Ekstrom K, Bossios A, Sjostrand M, Lee JJ, Lotvall JO. Exosome-mediated transfer of mRNAs and micro RNAs is a novel mechanism of genetic exchange between cells. Nature Cell Biology. 2007;**9**(6):654-659

[105] Yang C, Robbins PD. Immunosuppressive exosomes: A new approach for treating arthritis. International Journal of Rheumatology. 2012;**2012**:573528

[106] Cumpelik A, Ankli B, Zecher D, Schifferli JA. Neutrophil microvesicles resolve gout by inhibiting C5a-mediated priming of the inflammasome. Annals of the Rheumatic Diseases. 2016;**75**(6):1236-1245

[107] Saaf AM, Tengvall-Linder M, Chang HY, Adler AS, Wahlgren CF, Scheynius A, et al. Global expression profiling in atopic eczema reveals reciprocal expression of inflammatory and lipid genes. PLoS One. 2008;**3**(12):e4017

[108] Migita K, Koga T, Satomura K, Izumi M, Torigoshi T, Maeda Y, et al. Serum amyloid A triggers the mosodium urate-mediated mature interleukin-1beta production from human synovial fibroblasts. Arthritis Research & Therapy. 2012;**14**(3):R119

[109] Turnbaugh PJ, Ley RE, Hamady M, Fraser-Liggett CM, Knight R, Gordon JI. The human microbiome project. Nature. 2007;**449**(7164):804-810

[110] Cox MJ, Cookson WO, Moffatt MF. Sequencing the human microbiome in health and disease. Human Molecular Genetics. 2013;**22**(R1):R88-R94

[111] Guo Z, Zhang J, Wang Z, Ang KY, Huang S, Hou Q, et al. Intestinal microbiota distinguish gout patients from healthy humans. Scientific Reports. 2016;**6**:20602

[112] Albrecht E, Waldenberger M, Krumsiek J, Evans AM, Jeratsch U, Breier M, et al. Metabolite profiling reveals new insights into the regulation of serum urate in humans. Metabolomics: Official Journal of the Metabolomic Society. 2014;**10**(1):141-151

[113] Becker KG, Barnes KC, Bright TJ, Wang SA. The genetic association database. Nature Genetics. 2004;**36**(5):431-432

[114] Boks MP, Derks EM, Weisenberger DJ, Strengman E, Janson E, Sommer IE, et al. The relationship of DNA methylation with age, gender and genotype in twins and healthy controls. PLoS One. 2009;**4**(8):e6767

[115] Khanna D, Khanna PP, Fitzgerald JD, Singh MK, Bae S, Neogi T, et al. 2012 American College of Rheumatology guidelines for management of gout. Part 2: Therapy and antiinflammatory prophylaxis of acute gouty arthritis. Arthritis Care & Research. 2012;**64**(10):1447-1461

[116] Dalbeth N, Stamp LK, Merriman TR. The genetics of gout: Towards personalised medicine? BMC Medicine. 2017;**15**(1):108

[117] Batt C, Phipps-Green AJ, Black MA, Cadzow M, Merriman ME, Topless R, et al. Sugar-sweetened beverage consumption: A risk factor for prevalent gout with SLC2A9 genotype-specific effects on serum urate and risk of gout. Annals of the Rheumatic Diseases. 2014;**73**(12):2101-2106

[118] Hamajima N, Naito M, Okada R, Kawai S, Yin G, Morita E, et al. Significant interaction between LRP2 rs 2544390 in intron 1 and alcohol drinking for serum uric acid levels among a Japanese population. Gene. 2012;**503**(1):131-136

[119] Rasheed H, Phipps-Green A, Topless R, Hollis-Moffatt JE, Hindmarsh JH, Franklin C, et al. Association of the lipoprotein receptor-related protein 2 gene with gout and non-additive interaction with alcohol consumption. Arthritis Research & Therapy. 2013;**15**(6):R177

Chapter 5

Prophylaxis of Acute Arthritis at Initiation of Urate-Lowering Therapy in Gout Patients

Maxim Eliseev, Maria Chikina and Evgeny Nasonov

Abstract

During the first months after the initiation of urate-lowering therapy in gout patients, the risk of exacerbation of arthritis considerably rises, which often results in discontinuation of the prescribed therapy by patients. The main way to avoid this risk is preventive prescription of colchicine, NSAIDs or glucocorticoids. Such prophylaxis of acute arthritis has been specified in a large number of the latest editions of various national and international guidelines; however, this tactics is rarely used in practice. The chapter includes the most significant studies on this problem.

Keywords: gout, prophylaxis, urate-lowering therapy, NSAID, colchicine, GC, canakinumab, acute attack

1. Introduction

It is known that the frequency of gout attacks increases at initiation of any medications (allopurinol, febuxostat, PEG-uricase, and benzbromarone) that lower serum uric acid level, irrespectively of their mechanism of action [1, 2]. The most promising method to reduce the risk of acute arthritis in gout patients is to initiate preventive anti-inflammatory drug therapy (NSAIDs, colchicine, or glucocorticoids).

The need for preventive therapy of gout flares is also stated in the current guidelines [3, 4]. Thus, according to the guidelines by the European League against Rheumatism (EULAR), the need for prophylaxis of future gout flares should be explained to every patient and discussed with them. As the first-line therapy drug, it is recommended to use 0.5–1.0 mg colchicine daily and the dose should be lowered if the patient was diagnosed with renal insufficiency. Besides, the authors of the guidelines emphasize the need for observing the patients with renal insufficiency who receive HMG-CoA reductase inhibitors (statins) at the initiation of colchicine, considering the potential risks of neuro- and/or muscle toxicity. According to the guidelines, simultaneous prescription of colchicine and strong P-glycoprotein inhibitors and/or CYP3A4 should be avoided. In cases of intolerance to colchicine or contraindications for thereof, it is advised to consider prophylaxis with NSAID (also in the minimum effective anti-inflammatory dose, with the use of gastroprotective therapy if needed) [3]. The guidelines by the American College of Rheumatology (ACR) are similar to those by EULAR, however, according to the

IntechOpen

Source (study)	Type of study/trial	Drug	Period of observation	Number of patients	Results
Paulus et al., 1974 [9]	Double-blind placebo-controlled	Colchicine 0.5 mg 3 times daily	6 months	38	• The patients who received probenecid with colchicine had on average 0.19 gout flares per month, whereas in the patients who received probenecid and placebo, the frequency of attacks was on average 0.48 per month.
Borstad et al., 2004 [1]	Double-blind placebo-controlled	Colchicine 0.6 mg twice per day	6 months	43	• The patients who had colchicine therapy reported of acute arthritis much less often (0.52 vs. 2.91, $p = 0.008$), and in the case of development of acute arthritis, the intensity of pain at VAS was lower (3.64 vs. 5.08, $p = 0.018$).
Karimzadeh et al., 2006 [10]	Randomized without placebo control	Colchicine 1 mg daily	1 year	229	• Basing on the received data, the researchers came to the conclusion that the optimal length of colchicine therapy for prophylaxis of acute arthritis is 7–9 months from the start of urate-lowering therapy.
Wortmann et al., 2010 [38]	Randomized placebo-controlled	Colchicine 0.6 mg daily or naproxen 250 mg twice a day	6 months	4101	• In the groups where patients received colchicine or NSAIDs, they reported of reduction of the frequency of acute arthritis during the entire period of therapy, irrespectively of the selected medication. • Immediately after discontinuation of the 8-week prophylactic therapy, the frequency of acute arthritis increased by three times, irrespectively of the drug used for prophylaxis.
Jinquan et al., 2018 [45]	Comparative retrospective placebo-controlled	Colchicine 0.53 ± 0.15 mg daily or prednisolone 7.55 ± 1.3 mg daily	6 months	273	• Gout flares were noted more often in the patients who received therapy with prednisolone. • However, the intensity of pain during the acute arthritis was higher in the patients who received colchicine.
Schlesinger et al., 2011 [47]	Double-blind randomized active-controlled	Canakinumab 10, 25, 50, 90, 150 mg, one-time or triamcinolone acetonide (TA) 40 mg, one-time	8 weeks	200	• The reduction in pain on the canakinumab therapy was more marked than on TA in 25, 48 and 72 hours. • The period between gout flares on canakinumab was longer than on TA.
Schlesinger et al., 2012 [48]	Double-blind randomized multicenter controlled	Canakinumab 150 mg, one-time or triamcinolone acetonide (TA) 40 mg, one-time	24 weeks	465	• Reduction of the risk of gouty arthritis attacks by 66% in 12 weeks. • Reduction of the average number of new gouty arthritis attacks by 63% in 12 weeks.
Solomon et al., 2018 [49]	Randomized placebo-controlled	Canakinumab 50 mg, 150 or 300 mg once in 3 months	3.7 years	10,061	• Quarterly reception of canakinumab allowed to significantly reduce the risk of acute arthritis, irrespectively of the serum uric acid level.

Table 1.
Efficacy of prophylactic anti-inflammatory therapy at initiation of urate-lowering drugs in gout patients.

latter, in cases of contraindications for NSAID and colchicine, it is possible to initiate low-dose glucocorticoids [4].

Such prophylaxis is recommended to be given for 6 months from the start of urate-lowering therapy. This exact tactic allows to not only minimize the risk of acute arthritis, but also to reduce probability of self-discontinuation of the urate-lowering therapy by the patient.

However, the evidence basis for these recommendations is not ample and there have been no randomized controlled comparative trials of certain medications.

The most considerable studies on preventive anti-inflammatory therapy at the start of urate-lowering drug therapy are presented in **Table 1**.

2. Colchicine

Colchicine, an alkaloid received from *Colchicum autumnale*, is the most well-studied medication used for prophylaxis of acute arthritis at the initiation of urate-lowering therapy [5].

The mechanisms by which colchicine has its anti-inflammatory action are manifold. Probably the most valuable of these mechanisms is the effect on tubulin molecule, which conditions its cytotoxic and anti-inflammatory action due to the inhibition of migration, chemotaxis, neutrophil adhesion, as well as the suppression of superoxide anion synthesis [5].

The modern data suggest the possibility of the direct anti-inflammatory action of colchicine associated with IL-1-stimulated neutrophil adhesion inhibition. It has been recently shown that colchicine reducing pro-caspase-1 mRNA and secreted caspase-1 protein, an enzymatic component of NLR of the NOD-like receptor Pirin-3 (NLRP3) which regulates conversion of pro-interleukin-1β (IL-1β) into active IL-1β [6].

In 1961, Yu and Gutman first performed a study to estimate the possibility to use low-dose colchicine for exacerbation prophylaxis, which resulted in reduction of the frequency of acute arthritis both in the patients who received colchicine mono therapy and in those who received colchicine with concurrent probenecid. The duration of the therapy was 2–10 years, the patients received 0.5–2.0 mg colchicine daily, which was less than the colchicine dose typically used for rapid relief from acute arthritis at that time. As a result, the frequency and severity of acute arthritis considerably reduced in 74% patients; there were no differences in the frequency in the groups of patients who received probenecid and of those who did not, and the discontinuation of colchicine caused arthritis exacerbation within several weeks or months in 20 out of 25 patients who had not had acute arthritis for several years [7].

In 1965, Gutman published the findings of a retrospective analysis of 734 gout patients in which it was stated that reception of colchicine significantly reduced frequency of acute arthritis, irrespectively of the chosen urate-lowering therapy [8].

The first placebo-controlled study to show the efficacy of colchicine prophylaxis in acute gout arthritis was the study by Paulus et al. [9]. The study involved 51 gout patients with typical gout flares and serum uric acid level of >7.5 mg/dl. The patients were randomized and divided into two groups: probenecid 500 mg and colchicine 0.5 mg three times daily, or probenecid 500 mg and a placebo three times daily. The analysis included 38 patients who showed significant reduction in their average serum uric acid level. During the study, the patients reported about gout attacks which were classified as light, moderate and severe, and only those classified as moderate and severe were included in the analysis. As a result, during the study period, the patients from the probenecid/colchicine group had on average 0.19 gout attacks per month, while the patients from the probenecid/placebo group reported about on average 0.48 attacks per month.

In 2004, Borstad et al. [1] carried out the first study to evaluate the efficacy of low-dose colchicine at initiation of urate-lowering therapy (allopurinol). The study included 43 patients with established gout who began allopurinol therapy. As a gout flare prophylaxis, the patients took either colchicine 0.6 mg twice a day or a placebo, depending on their randomization. Both groups were analogous in their basic characteristics and in the doses of allopurinol necessary to reach the target uric acid level. The observation period was 6 months. The patients who took colchicine reported about gout flares much less often (0.52 vs. 2.91, $p = 0.008$), and in the cases of development of gout flares, the intensity of pain according to VAS was lower (3.64 vs. 5.08, $p = 0.018$). The tolerance of colchicine was good, however, the frequency of diarrhea was higher in the patients who took colchicine (38.0% in the colchicine patients vs. 4.5% in the placebo patients), and the reduction of the dose of colchicine to 0.6 mg once a day leveled those differences almost completely.

The study by Karimzadeh et al. [10] estimated the optimal length of colchicine therapy for prophylaxis of acute arthritis in gout patients. 229 patients using the allopurinol and colchicine 1 mg daily therapy were randomized into three groups: group 1 took colchicine for 3–6 months, group 2 for 7–9 months and group 3 for 10–12 months. After a one-year observation period, 54% of the patients in group 1, 27.5% of the patients in group 2, and 23% of the patients in group 3 had at least one gout flare. Basing on the received data, it was concluded that the optimal length of colchicine treatment for prophylaxis is 7–9 months. However, that study had a number of limitations as it was not placebo-controlled, the patients only informed about the time interval until the flare, not about the number of flares. Besides, the study did not provide any information on which criteria had been used to diagnose gout. Another important limitation of this study, just like of many others, was absence of a clear definition of gout flare for self-assessment by the patient. Recently the results of a multicenter work have been published which compared several simple ways of self-assessment which, as is expected, can reduce the possibility of making mistakes in investigation findings [11].

It is proved that bioavailability of colchicine is the same for elderly and young people. However, the distribution volume of colchicine can go down, which leads to its higher concentration in plasma and a significantly higher risk of toxicity. To counteract this effect, some experts recommend reducing the dose of colchicine by two times in the patients over 70 years old [12].

Critics of long reception of colchicine for gout flare prophylaxis at the start of urate-lowering therapy discuss how safe this tactics of therapy is. The doses of colchicine of 0.5–0.8 mg/kg are highly toxic and the doses over 0.8 mg/kg are usually fatal; in order to reduce the risk of irreversible overdose, the US Food and Drug Administration called off the permission to use colchicine intravenously [13]. Acute overdose of colchicine usually appears as gastrointestinal symptoms within 24 hours after taking, multiple organ failure (renal insufficiency, circulatory deficiency, bone marrow destruction, muscle weakness, rhabdomyolysis, and respiratory failure) within 7 days, and finally ends up with either resolution of symptoms or progression of dysfunction of organs and eventual death [14–17].

Chronic overdose of colchicine can arise when daily doses of colchicine are not adjusted for renal insufficiency or simultaneous reception of certain medications; colchicine neuromyopathy and cytopenia are classical characteristics of chronic overdose [14].

Colchicine predominantly binds three proteins: tubulin, Cytochrome P3A4 (CYP3A4) and P-glycoprotein (Pgp) [18].

CYP3A4 is contained in hepatocytes and enterocytes and metabolizes colchicine to 2.3 dimethyl colchicine. P-glycoprotein, which is contained in enterocytes, hepatocytes, renal and other cells, limits gastrointestinal absorption of colchicine.

Along with renal excretion, these systems determine general level of colchicine in blood serum. Individual content of CYP3A4 and P-glycoprotein conditions absence of adequate response to colchicine in some patients, which can be associated with excessive expression of one or both of these proteins [19]. CYP3A4 and P-glycoprotein are also responsible for interaction between colchicine and other medications. Because of its interaction with CYP3A4, colchicine can have harmful effect if simultaneously taken with clarithromycin, fluoxetine, paroxetine and other inhibitors of proteases, which are metabolized with the aid of this ferment [20].

Several descriptions of clinical cases and one retrospective review show that combination of colchicine and inhibitors of HMG-CoA reductase, which also interact with CYP3A4, can sometimes increase the risk of acute myopathy [21–23].

Kuritzky and Panchal debate about advisability and safety of prophylactic reception of anti-inflammatory medications at the start of urate-lowering therapy, referring to a large number of adverse drug reactions in such a therapy [24]. Under discussion is the possibility for the patient to choose between constant therapy during average 6 months or rapid relief of flares as required. Also, the authors came to the conclusion that long use of colchicine is safer than that of NSAIDs. It was noted that myopathy and rhabdomyolysis are registered more often in the cases of high doses and simultaneous use with not only HMG-CoA reductase inhibitors (statins) but also with fibrates, verapamil, diltiazem, cyclosporine and others, which presupposes the need for serious control in case of their simultaneous use.

Kuncl et al. [14] presented a description of 12 new cases of typical syndromes of myopathy and neuropathy amid use of colchicine by gout patients. Myopathy usually appears as proximal weakness and is always accompanied by higher serum level of creatine kinase; both appearances remain for at least 3 or 4 weeks after discontinuation of the medication. Accompanying axonal polyneuropathy is usually mild, but resolves slowly after discontinuation. Electromyography of proximal muscles usually reveals myopathy which is characterized by abnormal spontaneous activity. Due to these peculiarities, c-induced myopathy is often diagnosed incorrectly, either as probable polymyositis or uremic neuropathy. C-induced myopathy is characterized by accumulation of lysosomes and autophagosomes unrelated to necrosis or moderate denervation in distal muscles. Morphological changes in muscles indicate that pathogenesis relates to damage of microtubular cytoskeletal network which interacts with lysosomes. Correct diagnosis can save patients with such a disorder from a wrong therapy. Myotoxicity most often arises in people over 50–70 years old who take 1.2 mg colchicine daily. Thus, prescription of a long-term colchicine therapy for patients over 50 years old should be carried out with maximal caution.

Tolerance to colchicine is dose-dependent and the recommended dose for prophylaxis of arthritis (0.6 mg once or twice a day), as a rule, is better tolerable than higher doses used earlier to treat acute gout arthritis (1.2 mg at acute flare with subsequent increase by 0.6 mg hourly) [25]. The most common colchicine-induced adverse drug reactions occur with the gastrointestinal tract, namely nausea and diarrhea, which are reported by 5–10% of the patients, even in cases of low-dose colchicine [26]. Gastrotoxicity is highly likely to depend on the dose and can be reduced by decreasing the dose of colchicine.

Among other adverse drug reactions related to the toxicity of colchicine, we should note neuropathy [24], cytopenia (thrombo-, leuko-, pancytopenia, and aplastic anemia), disseminated intravascular coagulation and metabolic acidosis [27, 28].

Fortunately, probability of adverse drug reactions is low, nevertheless in cases of long-term treatment with colchicine it is necessary to perform regular analysis of clinical blood test, level of creatine phosphokinase, transaminases, which is particularly important in elderly patients, especially in cases of simultaneous reception of some of the abovementioned medications.

Besides the possibility of prophylaxis of acute gout flares at the initiation of urate-lowering medications and titration of their dose, there have been discussions about the favorable effect of colchicine on the cardiovascular system [29]. Retrospective cohort studies in patients with gout report a lower incidence of combined cardiovascular outcomes in those treated with colchicine [30].

Thus, in the retrospective crossover study Crittenden et al. [31] investigated whether use of colchicine relates to reduction of risk of myocardial infarction (MI) in gout patients. The primary outcome was diagnostication of MI, the secondary outcomes included all-cause mortality and C-reactive protein (CRP) level. Altogether 1288 patients were diagnosed with gout. The groups of patients who received colchicine ($n = 576$) and of those who did not ($n = 712$) were comparable in demographic criteria and their serum uric acid level. Prevalence of MI was 1.2% in the group who received colchicine, as against 2.6% in the group who did not ($p = 0.03$).

In the next study it was proved that reception of 0.5 mg of colchicine daily in addition to the therapy with statins and other medications used for secondary prevention of cardiovascular catastrophes, led to reduction of cases of development of acute coronary syndrome, out-of-hospital cardiac arrest and ischemic stroke [hazard ratio (HR) 0.33; 95% confidence interval (CI) 0.18–0.59; $p < 0.001$] [32].

Meta-analysis of trials of colchicine in multiple cardiovascular diseases revealed a decrease in myocardial infarction with varying levels of evidence [30].

Currently the randomized controlled CONVINCE trial is enrolling stroke patients to evaluate the effect of a daily low-dose of colchicine in reducing the rate of recurrent stroke and major vascular events [33].

3. NSAIDs

Along with colchicine, NSAIDs are used as the first line drug therapy for acute arthritis prophylaxis in gout patients. Just like with colchicine, the history of using NSAIDs for gout is centuries old. Thus, among the ancestors of the modern anti-inflammatory drugs there were vegetable foods containing salicylic acid, such as willow bark, meadowsweet, dried raspberries and others [34–36].

At present, there are no works which could determine the optimal dose or duration of NSAIDs treatment for prophylaxis of acute gout arthritis [37].

Within the frameworks of phase 3 trial on comparison of efficacy of inhibitors of xanthine oxidase of allopurinol and febuxostat, the effect of low-dose colchicine therapy on the frequency of acute arthritis during the first weeks of urate-lowering therapy was assessed. Selection of a certain drug for prophylaxis of acute arthritis was performed directly by the doctor. In 79.6% cases they chose colchicine in the dose of 0.6 mg daily, in 15.2% cases—NSAIDs (naproxen 250 mg twice a day), and the remaining 5.1% patients did not receive prophylactic treatment. In the groups where the patients took colchicine or NSAIDs, the frequency of gout attacks during the entire period of treatment reduced, irrespectively of the medication. It is interesting that immediately after the discontinuation of the 8-week prophylactic therapy, the frequency of gout attacked increased by three times irrespectively of which medication was used for prophylaxis and remained higher than the original during several months of treatment with both xanthine oxidase inhibitors. The frequency of unfavorable effects of colchicine treatment (55.1%) was higher than that of naproxen (44.3%) ($p < 0.001$), however, colchicine was used more often (selection of the medication was carried out by the researcher, without randomization), and in the case of decrease of creatinine clearance <50 ml/min naproxen was not prescribed [38].

These facts explains limitation of long-term use of NSAIDs. Firstly, it relates to the increase in the frequency of NSAIDs-related adverse drug reactions from the gastrointestinal tract [39]. Secondly, to the need of a considerable part of gout patients for acetylsalicylic acid medications.

Besides, NSAIDs should be used with caution in gout patients with lower glomerular filtration rate (long use of NSAIDs by such patients is contraindicated) because they can lead to acute and chronic renal insufficiency, nephrotic syndrome with interstitial nephritis, papillary necrosis, lower clearance of potassium and sodium [40].

In 2010, a study was carried out to assess efficacy of urate-lowering therapy with allopurinol and febuxostat. During the period from February 2010 to December 2010, 516 out of 679 respondents were randomly (1:1:1) prescribed febuxostat 40, 80 mg or allopurinol 300 mg. As prophylactic anti-inflammatory therapy, the patients, during the first 8 weeks, received 0.5 mg of colchicine daily or 7.5 mg of meloxicam daily. As a result, the number of patients who needed treatment of acute gout attacks from the 9th to the 28th week was extremely low: 4.07% (7/172) in the group on 80 mg febuxostat, 5.23% (9/172) in the group on 40 mg febuxostat and 9.3% (16/172) in the group on allopurinol. Besides the considerable reduction of the number of acute attacks during the urate-lowering therapy in all groups, the study revealed high adherence of patients and low percentage of patients who discontinued urate-lowering therapy (on average 5%), which often related to development of unfavorable reactions [41].

Use of NSAIDs also related to increased risk of cardiovascular pathology, which makes it even harder to choose a certain medication because every other gout patient has a high risk of cardiovascular complications [42].

4. Glucocorticoids

In case of impossibility to prescribe NSAIDs or colchicine and/or their inefficacy for prophylaxis of acute arthritis in gout patients, it is proposed to prescribe low-dose glucocorticoids, however, there is little data on their long-term therapy in gout patients [43].

It is thought that prescription of low-dose prednisolone can be efficient and safer than NSAIDs for treatment of acute arthritis in gout patients. However, there have been no randomized controlled trials aimed at investigating comparative efficacy of glucocorticoids and NSAIDs [44].

So far, the first and only comparative study of efficacy of colchicine and glucocorticoids at the initiation of urate-lowering therapy, namely febuxostat therapy, is the study by Yu et al. [45]. The study included 273 patients, where 152 patients received colchicine as acute arthritis prophylactic therapy, 49 received prednisolone, and the remaining 72 patients did not receive any anti-inflammatory medications. The mean daily dosage of febuxostat in the groups of patients receiving colchicine, glucocorticoids and in the control group was 41.97 ± 10.74, 40.82 ± 9.09, and 41.67 ± 9.93 mg daily respectively. The mean daily dosage of colchicine was 0.53 ± 0.15 mg daily, the duration of therapy 6.13 ± 1.14 months. The mean daily dosage of prednisolone was 7.55 ± 1.30 mg daily, the duration of therapy was 6.20 ± 1.36 months. The target serum uric acid level of <360 μmol/l was achieved in each group. No severe ADRs were noted. The analysis of the data showed that acute arthritis attacks were reported 271 times altogether, where 46 attacks (21.7%) in the colchicine group, 47 (44.9%) in the glucocorticoids group and 178 (91.7%) in the control group. However, at high frequency of recurrent gouty arthritis, the intensity of pain during acute arthritis was lower in the patients who received glucocorticoids therapy.

5. Canakinumab

A considerable part of gout patients have contraindications for NSAID, colchicine and glucocorticoids, and often such therapy can be ineffective, especially in patients with severe tophaseous gout, which implies the need for using other methods of therapy. For such patients, it is advisable to consider the use of IL-1 inhibitors, at least the use of long half-life medications (in particular IL-1β: canakinumab).

Among possible methods of prophylaxis, use of IL-1 inhibitors can be discussed, at least use of medications with long half-life (in particular IL-1β: canakinumab). Use of the medication in gout patients is limited to solely rapid relief of arthritis resistant to any other anti-inflammatory therapy or in case of its impossibility. However, the steady anti-inflammatory effect of the medication, which surpasses that of both colchicine and glucocorticoids, allows to initiate therapy with urate-lowering drugs and perform titration of the dose of allopurinol with minimal risk of development of acute arthritis [46, 47].

Within the framework of a 24-week phase 2 trial, the efficacy of different doses of canakinumab and colchicine was compared in 432 gout patients [46]. The plans of therapy determined by randomization included subcutaneous injections of 25, 50, 100, 200 or 300 mg of canakinumab on the first day or four injections with four-week intervals (50 mg on the first day and in the fourth week and 25 mg on the eighth and twelfth weeks) or daily reception of colchicine 0.5 mg per os daily during 16 weeks. It was established that the average number of gout attacks was lower with any dose of canakinumab, with maximal of 100–300 mg. In the cases of the use of canakinumab doses of ≥50 mg, the average number of attacks was lower by 62–72% than in the case of colchicine, and the risk of at least one attack was lower by 64–72%.

The two following 12-week double-blind multicenter controlled trials of phase 3 carried out with the same design and united for analysis (β-RELIEVED and β-RELIEVED II) compared the efficacy of 150 mg canakinumab and 40 mg triamcinolone acetonide (TA) as a means of prophylaxis of acute arthritis [48]. Canakinumab significantly increased the period between attacks and reduced the risk of recurrent gouty arthritis (by 63% in 12 weeks and by 56% in 24 weeks). Moreover, the median time period between attacks for canakinumab was 168 days, which exceeded the duration of the trial (24 weeks).

In their study Solomon et al. [49] compared the frequency of gout attacks at the initiation of urate-lowering therapy in patients with different original serum uric acid levels (≤404.5, 404.6–535.3, and ≥ 535.4 μmol/l). As prophylaxis of gout flares they used canakinumab in different doses (50, 150, and 300 mg), which was injected subcutaneously every 3 months. The observation period was almost 4 years and after analyzing the received data it was found that quarterly injection of canakinumab was associated with a significantly lower risk of acute arthritis, irrespectively of the serum uric acid level.

Canakinumab therapy is generally well-tolerated, although all the studies associated the use of canakinumab with the increase in infectious adverse drug reactions (ADR), including severe ones. The probability of ADR was comparable for any of the used doses of canakinumab (51.9–58.5%) and colchicine (53.7%) [46]. Most of the ADR were light or moderate, and severe ADR were registered in 14 (4.3%) patients receiving canakinumab and six (5.6%) patients receiving colchicine. All six cases of severe ADR in four patients were registered in the canakinumab group. In another phase 2 trial, the total frequency of ADR was also comparable (41.3% in the canakinumab group and 42.1% in the TA group) with the frequency of severe ADR (2.8 and 1.8% respectively) [50]. The only case of infectious bronchitis was registered in the canakinumab group, but, from the researchers' point of view, it was unlikely to be associated with the reception of the drug. Finally, in the phase 3 trials united for the analysis, where the dose of canakinumab was one-time 150 mg, the differences in the frequency of ADR (66.2% in the canakinumab group and 52.8% in the TA group) were conditioned by infectious ADR, mainly non-severe infections of upper airways (20.4% in the canakinumab group and 12.2% in the TA group) [48].

None of the studies registered fatal cases associated with infectious diseases. Although the use of canakinumab was accompanied by moderate reduction of the levels of thrombocytes, leucocytes and neutrophils in the blood, it did not have clinical relevance.

Canakinumab therapy should be carried out by a rheumatologist experienced in gout treatment and genetically biological disease modifying antirheumatic drugs (bDMARDs). Before the start of the therapy, it is important to exclude active and latent tuberculosis infections. The recommended dose of canakinumab is 150 mg (subcutaneously). If there is need for a repeated injection, the interval between the two should be over 12 weeks. In case of no effect after the first injection, it is inadvisable to give repeated injections.

6. Conclusion

To summarize, it should be noted that neglect of recommendations on prophylaxis of acute arthritis during the first months of urate-lowering therapy, despite the

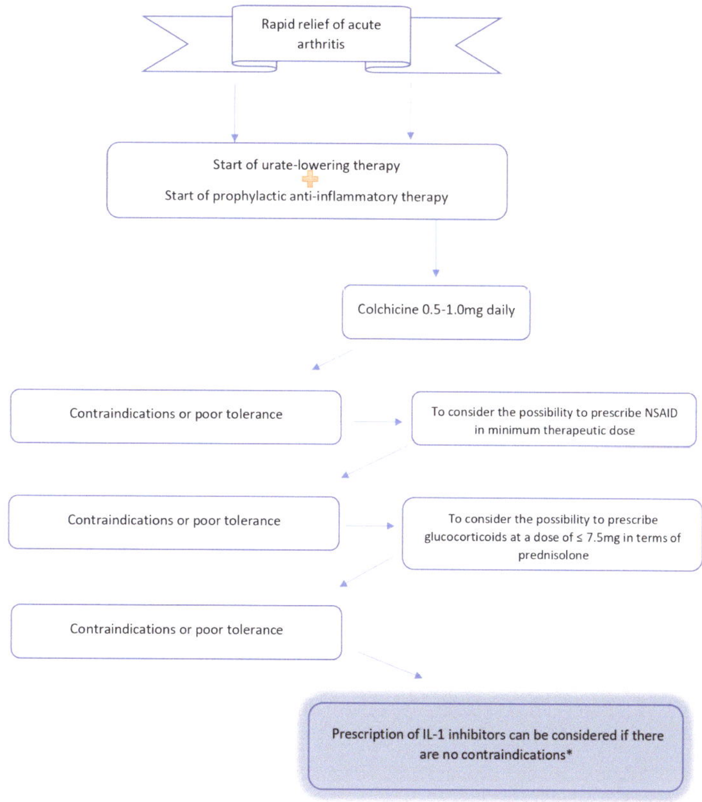

Figure 1.
*Acute arthritis prophylaxis algorithm at initiation of urate-lowering therapy in gout patients. *There are no recommendations for use of canakinumab for prophylaxis of acute arthritis, however, it can be effective at initiation of urate-lowering therapy in patients with severe tophaceous gout and frequent gout flares [48, 49].*

firm guidelines of its necessity, is one of the most common mistakes in treatment of gout [51]. For example, according to the analysis of the database of 643 gout patients who were first prescribed allopurinol, only 26% were also prescribed prophylactic anti-inflammatory therapy (16% received NSAIDs and 10%—colchicine) [52]. At that, besides the burden of pain and poorer working ability which result from acute arthritis, this exact mistake can be the main cause of patient's discontinuation of urate-lowering medications and patient's low adherence to treatment. As a result—development of chronic arthritis, formation of tophi, as well as gouty arthropathy and bone tissue destruction. One of the ways to avoid the above said is to adhere to the recommendations on gout treatment whose integral part is prophylaxis of acute arthritis at the initiation of urate-lowering medications. The suggested algorithm of the drug prophylaxis of acute arthritis during the first months of urate-lowering therapy presupposes sequential selection of the anti-inflammatory medication (see **Figure 1**). As the first-line medication, it is advised to use colchicine, in cases of contraindications for or poor tolerance to thereof—NSAID, and if NSAID therapy is not possible either—glucocorticoids. Finally, for the patients with chronic arthritis and the need for regular use of anti-inflammatory drugs, it is possible to consider IL-1 inhibitors (canakinumab).

Author details

Maxim Eliseev*, Maria Chikina and Evgeny Nasonov
V.A. Nasonova Research Institute of Rheumatology, Moscow, Russia

*Address all correspondence to: elicmax@rambler.ru

References

[1] Borstad GC, Bryant LR, Abel MP, et al. Colchicine for prophylaxis of acute flares when initiating allopurinol for chronic gouty arthritis. The Journal of Rheumatology. 2004;**31**:2429-2432

[2] Sarawate CA, Patel PA, Schumacher HR, et al. Serum urate levels and gout flares: Analysis from managed care data. Journal of Clinical Rheumatology. 2006;**12**(2):61-65

[3] Richette P, Doherty M, Pascual E, Barskova V. 2016 updated EULAR evidence-based recommendations for the management of gout. Annals of the Rheumatic Diseases. 2017;**76**(1):29-42

[4] Khanna D, Khanna PP, Fitzgerald JD, et al. American College of Rheumatology guidelines for management of gout. Part 2: Therapy and antiinflammatory prophylaxis of acute gouty arthritis. Arthritis Care & Research (Hoboken). 2012;**64**:1447-1461

[5] Terkeltaub RA. Colchicine update: 2008. Seminars in Arthritis and Rheumatism. 2009;**38**(6):411-419

[6] Robertson S, Martínez GJ, Payet CA, et al. Colchicine therapy in acute coronary syndrome patients acts on caspase-1 to suppress NLRP3 inflammasome monocyte activation. Clinical Science (London, England). 2016;**130**(14):1237-1246

[7] Yu TF, Gutman AB. Efficacy of colchicine prophylaxis in gout. Prevention of recurrent gouty arthritis over a mean period of five years in 208 gouty subjects. Annals of Internal Medicine. 1961;**55**:179-192

[8] Gutman AB. Treatment of primary gout: The present status. Arthritis and Rheumatism. 1965;**8**:911-920

[9] Paulus HE, Schlosstein LH, Godfrey RG, et al. Prophylactic colchicine therapy of intercritical gout. A placebo-controlled study of probenecid treated patients. Arthritis and Rheumatism. 1974;**17**:609-614

[10] Karimzadeh H, Nazari J, Mottaghi P, Kabiri P. Different duration of colchicine for preventing recurrence of gouty arthritis. Journal of Research in Medical Sciences: The Official Journal of Isfahan University of Medical Sciences. 2006;**11**:104-107

[11] Gaffo AL, Singh JA, Dalbeth N, et al. Brief report: Validation of a definition of flare in patients with established gout. Arthritis & Rheumatology. 2018;**70**(3):462-467

[12] Rochdi M, Sabouraud A, Girre C, et al. Pharmacokinetics and absolute bioavailability of colchicine after i.v. and oral administration in healthy human volunteers and elderly subjects. Journal of Clinical Pharmacology. 1994;**46**(4):351-354

[13] Finkelstein Y, Aks SE, Hutson JR, et al. Colchicine poisoning: The dark side of an ancient drug. Clinical Toxicology (Philadelphia, Pa.). 2010;**48**(5):407-414

[14] Kuncl RW, Duncan G, Watson D, et al. Colchicine myopathy and neuropathy. The New England Journal of Medicine. 1987;**316**(25):1562-1568

[15] Mullins ME, Carrico EA, Horowitz BZ. Fatal cardiovascular collapse following acute colchicine ingestion. Journal of Toxicology. Clinical Toxicology. 2000;**38**(1):51-54

[16] Aghabiklooei A, Zamani N, Hassanian-Moghaddam H, et al. Acute colchicine overdose: Report of three cases. Reumatismo. 2013;**65**(6):307-311

[17] Yousuf Bhat Z, Reddy S, Pillai U, et al. Colchicine-induced myopathy

in a tacrolimus-treated renal transplant recipient: Case report and literature review. American Journal of Therapeutics. 2016;**23**(2):e614-e616

[18] Slobodnick A, Shah B, Michael H, et al. Colchicine: Old and new. The American Journal of Medicine. 2015;**128**(5):461-470

[19] Niel E, Scherrmann J-M. Colchicine today. Joint, Bone, Spine. 2006;**73**(6):672-678

[20] Cronstein BN, Sunkureddi P. Mechanistic aspects of inflammation and clinical management of inflammation in acute gouty arthritis. Journal of Clinical Rheumatology. 2013;**19**(1):19-29

[21] Frydrychowicz C, Pasieka B, Pierer M, Mueller W, Petros S, Weidhase L. Colchicine triggered severe rhabdomyolysis after long-term low-dose simvastatin therapy: A case report. Journal of Medical Case Reports. 2017;**11**(1):8

[22] Alayli G, Cengiz K, Cantürk F, Durmuş D, Akyol Y, Menekşe EB. Acute myopathy in a patient with concomitant use of pravastatin and colchicine. The Annals of Pharmacotherapy. 2005;**39**(7-8):1358-1361

[23] Hsu WC, Chen WH, Chang MT, Chiu HC. Colchicine-induced acute myopathy in a patient with concomitant use of simvastatin. Clinical Neuropharmacology. 2002;**25**(5):266-268

[24] Kuritzky L, Panchal R. Gout: Nonsteroidal anti-inflammatory drugs and colchicine to prevent painful flares during early uratelowering therapy. Journal of Pain & Palliative Care Pharmacotherapy. 2010;**24**(4):397-401

[25] Yang LP. Oral colchicine (Colcrys®) in the treatment and prophylaxis of gout: Profile report. Drugs & Aging. 2010;**27**(10):855-857

[26] Angelidis C, Kotsialou Z, Kossyvakis C, et al. Colchicine pharmacokinetics and mechanism of action. Current Pharmaceutical Design. 2018;**24**(6):659-663

[27] Singh J, Yang S, Foster J. The risk of aplastic anemia and pancytopenia with colchicine: A retrospective study of integrated health system database. Arthritis and Rheumatism. 2014;**66**(11):20

[28] Stanley MW, Taurog JD, Snover DC. Fatal colchicine toxicity: Report of a case. Clinical and Experimental Rheumatology. 1984;**2**(2):167-171

[29] Hansson GK. Inflammation, atherosclerosis, and coronary artery disease. The New England Journal of Medicine. 2005;**352**:1685-1695

[30] Fiolet ATL, Nidorf SM, Mosterd A, Cornel JH. Colchicine in stable coronary artery disease. Clinical Therapeutics. 2018;**pii**:S0149-2918(18)30462-4

[31] Crittenden DB, Lehmann RA, Schneck L, et al. Colchicine use is associated with decreased prevalence of myocardial infarction in patients with gout. The Journal of Rheumatology. 2012;**39**:1458-1464

[32] Nidorf S, Eikelboom J, Budgeon C, et al. Low-dose colchicine for secondary prevention of cardiovascular disease. Journal of the American College of Cardiology. 2013;**61**:404-410

[33] Gulati S, Dubois P, Carter B, Gulati S, Dubois P, Carter B, et al. A randomized crossover trial of conventional vs virtual chromoendoscopy for colitis surveillance: Dysplasia detection, feasibility, and patient acceptability (CONVINCE). Inflammatory Bowel Diseases. 2018;**10**(10):1-11. DOI: 10.1093/ibd/izy360

[34] Vane J. The fight against rheumatism: From willow bark

to COX-1 sparing drugs. Journal of Physiology and Pharmacology. 2000;**51**(4 Pt 1):573-586

[35] Hebbes C, Lambert D. Non-opioid analgesics. Anaesthesia and Intensive Care Medicine. 2011;**12**(2):69-72

[36] Brune K. The early history of non-opioid analgesics. Acute Pain. 1997;**1**:33-40

[37] Doghramji PP. Managing your patient with gout: A review of treatment options. Postgraduate Medicine. 2011;**123**(3):56-71

[38] Wortmann RL, Macdonald PA, Hunt B, Jackson RL. Effect of prophylaxis on gout flares after the initiation of urate-lowering therapy: Analysis of data from three phase III trials. Clinical Therapeutics. 2010;**32**(14):2386-2397

[39] Pham K, Hirschberg R. Global safety of coxibs and NSAIDs. Current Topics in Medicinal Chemistry. 2005;**5**(5):465-473

[40] Munar MY, Singh H. Drug dosing adjustments in patients with chronic kidney disease. American Family Physician. 2007;**75**(10):1487-1496

[41] Huang X, Du H, Gu J, et al. An allopurinol-controlled, multicenter, randomized, double-blind, parallel between-group, comparative study of febuxostat in Chinese patients with gout and hyperuricemia. International Journal of Rheumatic Diseases. 2014;**17**(6):679-686

[42] Trelle S, Reichenbach S, Wandel S, et al. Cardiovascular safety of non-steroidal antiinflammatory drugs: Network meta-analysis. BMJ. 2011;**342**:70-86

[43] Janssens HJ, Lucassen PL, Van de Laar FA, et al. Systemic corticosteroids for acute gout. Cochrane Database of Systematic Reviews. 2008;**16**(2):CD005521

[44] Yu J, Lu H, Zhou J, et al. Oral prednisolone versus non-steroidal anti-inflammatory drugs in the treatment of acute gout: A meta-analysis of randomized controlled trials. Inflammopharmacology. 2018;**26**(3):717-723

[45] Yu J, Qiu Q, Liang L, Yang X, Xu H. Prophylaxis of acute flares when initiating febuxostat for chronic gouty arthritis in a real-world clinical setting. Modern Rheumatology. 2018;**28**(2):339-344

[46] Schlesinger N, Mysler E, Lin H-Y, et al. Canakinumab reduces the risk of acute gouty arthritis flares during initiation of allopurinol treatment: Results of a double-blind, randomised study. Annals of the Rheumatic Diseases. 2011;**1264, 70**:1264-1271

[47] Schlesinger N, De Meulemeester MD, Pikhlak A, et al. Canakinumab relieves symptoms of acute flares and improves health-related quality of life in patients with difficult-to-treat gouty arthritis by suppressing inflammation: Results of a randomized, dose-ranging study. Arthritis Research & Therapy. 2011;**13**:R53

[48] Schlesinger N, Alten R, Bardin T, et al. Canakinumab for acute gouty arthritis in patients with limited treatment options: Results from two randomised, multicentre, active-controlled, double-blind trials and their initial extensions. Annals of the Rheumatic Diseases. 2012;**71**:1839-1848

[49] Solomon D, Robert J, et al. Relationship of interleukin-1Blockade with incident gout and serum uric acid levels. Annals of Internal Medicine. 2018;**169**(8):535-542

[50] So A, De MM, Pikhlak A, et al. Canakinumab for the treatment of

acute flares in difficult-to-treat gouty arthritis: Results of a multicenter, phase II, dose-ranging study. Arthritis and Rheumatism. 2010;**62**:3064-3076

[51] Singh JA, Hodges JS, Asch SM. Opportunities for improving medication use and monitoring in gout. Annals of the Rheumatic Diseases. 2009;**68**(8):1265-1270

[52] Mitha E, Schumacher HR, Fouche L, et al. Rilonacept for gout flare prevention during initiation of uric acid-lowering therapy: Results from the PRESURGE-2 international, phase 3, randomized, placebo-controlled trial. Rheumatology. 2013;**52**(7):1285-1292